Cool
Irish Names
for Babies

D1513876

Collins

Cool Irish Names for Babies

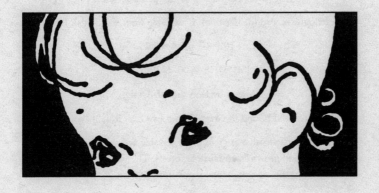

Pamela Redmond Satran

and

Linda Rosenkrantz

HarperCollins*Publishers*
77–85 Fulham Palace Road
London
W6 8JB

www.collins.co.uk

Collins is a registered trademark of HarperCollins Publishers Ltd.

First published in 2008

A catalogue record for this book is available from the British Library.

10 9 8 7 6 5 4 3 2 1

ISBN 978-0-00-727522-9

Typeset by Bob Vickers Design

Printed and bound in Great Britain by Clays Ltd, St Ives plc.

Collins uses papers that are natural, renewable and recyclable products
made from wood grown in sustainable forests. The manufacturing processes
conform to the environmental regulations of the country of origin.

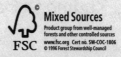

Mixed Sources
Product group from well-managed
forests and other controlled sources
www.fsc.org Cert no. SW-COC-1806
© 1996 Forest Stewardship Council

FSC is a non-profit international organisation established to promote the
responsible management of the world's forests. Products carrying the FSC
label are independently certified to assure consumers that they come
from forests that are managed to meet the social, economic and
ecological needs of present and future generations.

Find out more about HarperCollins and the environment at
www.harpercollins.co.uk/green

Contents

II. COOL COOL — Famous Names · 31

III. PRE-COOL COOL — Old Names · 67

IV. NEW COOL — Creative Names • 127

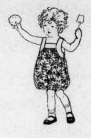

Introduction

What does cool mean when it comes to names for Irish babies? Something very different than it means for other kinds of baby names.

Our first edition of *Cool Names for Babies* was aimed at the American market, where cool names are often invented, drawn from a range of ethnic backgrounds, borrowed from places or surnames or things. In the USA, when it comes to baby names, anything from Heaven to Harlow to Harmony goes.

The British are more conservative, so when we devised the UK edition of *Cool Names*, we focused on the revival of such old-fashioned names as Edith and Arthur, on trendy short forms such as Dixie and Alfie, on royal names such as Leonie and Ludovic.

And then we came to the Irish. Irish baby-naming is a culture in itself, full of gorgeous and often obscure ancient names whose original bearers were kings and queens, mythological heroes and heroines, saints and fairies. During the centuries of British rule, these native Irish names were suppressed, with anglicised forms – Grace for Gráinne, Eugene for Eoghan – taking their place.

But after Irish independence, a priest named Patrick Woulfe started a campaign to restore the use of original Irish names. His 1923 book, *Irish Names for Children*, launched a national revolution in the way children were named. Ancient names were rediscovered, original forms were revived and a naming culture was restored to its original glory.

Today, such Irish names as Aoife and Conor and Niamh, Cian and Caoimhe and Cillian, Oisín and Róisín, Darragh and Aisling and Saoirse are at the top of the popularity charts. They share the spotlight with non-Irish names popular throughout the English-speaking world: Emma, Sophie and Ava for girls, Jack, Daniel and Luke for boys.

Which brings us back to the issue of cool.

Cool, when we're talking about Irish names, most often means traditional. In many ways what's old in Irish names *is* what's new. The coolest names these days are the most deeply rooted ones, spelt the original way. Names scrambling the fastest up the popularity ladder, for instance, include Fionn and Ruairí and Aoibhe (in tandem with Finn and Rory and Eve).

And if distinctive, undiscovered names often count for cool in the rest of the world, they do in Ireland as well, where the rosters are full of such treasures. You'll find them all in these pages, along with details about why their original bearers were so inspirational. Irish literature and theatre also offer a trove of stylish names with inspiring associations, along with lots of other sources, both expected and surprising.

Here are some basic rules to keep in mind when searching for a cool name for your baby:

Cool Means Unusual

In general, the more unusual a name, the cooler it is. With once-uncommon names such as Aoife, Luke and Ella now competing for the top spots, you have to move further and further from the mainstream to find a name that's truly distinctive. While fashionable Irish names such as Aisling and Cian may still be wonderful choices (and perhaps ultimately the right ones for you), you can't really call them cool. And trendy names ranging from Shane to Sophie, Chloe to Conor are simply too widely used to meet the prerequisites of cool.

Cool is Diverse

This is a trickier concept when it comes to names for Irish babies than it is for, say, American or British children, since the coolest names in Ireland are often the *least* diverse, the most ethnocentrically Irish. Still, Irish names don't have a monopoly on cool, and some Irish parents may wish to search farther afield for fresh choices. But you don't have to go too far: names from other Celtic cultures – Scottish and Welsh and Cornish and Breton – might provide the individuality you crave without sacrificing too much tradition. And if your tastes run more towards the pan-cultural Emma and Edward end of the spectrum, we've also included here names that are considered cool throughout the rest of an ever-shrinking Europe and across the Atlantic in the USA.

Cool Goes Beyond Convention

That's not to say there aren't fresh sources for Irish names with cultural resonance. Hero names – borne by politicians and poets and athletes – you might not have considered as first names are one idea. Irish last names are another, and not just the usual suspects such as Kelly and Ryan but O'Brien and Maguire and Sullivan as well. Irish place names can be yet another new locale in which to search for first names. And Irish words can be turned into names, too.

Cool Draws on Popular Culture

The world is full of inspiration for cool baby-naming – and more full every day, thanks to the innovative names of characters in films and books and to the names of star-babies and celebrities themselves. In these pages you'll find a rundown of the coolest names in modern Irish literature and film, and of the stars and their children who influence baby-naming style.

Don't Be Afraid of Cool

When today's parents were growing up, if you had an unusual name, other kids thought you were a bit odd. But now that the concept of cool permeates culture, with so many people from celebrities to the other kids in the classroom bearing unusual names, children are more apt to admire distinctive names than to ridicule them. Children today are often more accepting than adults of names that are unfamiliar, from different cultures or that cross gender lines.

There's More Than One Way to Be Cool

Cool wouldn't be cool if it was too regimented. There are cool names to suit any sensibility or level of cool, from the mainstream to the avant-garde. How far you want to go depends on your taste, your sense of adventure, your community. Before you settle at either end of the spectrum or on one particular name, weigh the various options and become comfortable with the brand and level of cool that fits you best.

Cool Isn't Everything

So what if you're one of those people who realise that a cool name isn't for you or your child? What if you read this book and find yourself intrigued, entertained, inspired… but in the end a lot more convinced than you realised that you want to give your child a plain, solid and decidedly uncool name such as John or Mary?

So what indeed. A name is not your personal style statement, a choice with which to impress the world. Rather, you should think of it as something that will identify your child for the rest of his or her life, a label he or she will have to live with forever. You may decide that cool is a desirable component of such a lifelong imprimatur. But then again, you may decide that, when it comes to a name, you want nothing to do with cool (just know you may have to suffer the consequences when your child is a teenager).

Whether or not you end up with a cool name, you owe it to your baby and your choice of a name to read this book. For one thing, you'll find hundreds and hundreds of naming options here that you won't find anywhere else, and that will open your eyes to a way of thinking about names that no other book or source can. And you'll know for certain, after reading this book, what constitutes a cool name – even if you eventually decide that uncool is cool enough for you.

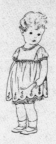

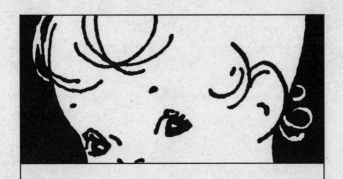

I. POP COOL

...

Mainstream Names

Aoife

Top of the Lists

For many people, Irish and others alike, there's nothing cooler than a popular name. The theory is that a popular name makes a child feel popular – accepted and approved – simply because he or she has a name that's familiar to all and currently in style. Here then, from the Central Statistics Office in Dublin, are the current Top 50 names in Ireland:

Boys

SEÁN	DANIEL
JACK	LUKE
CONOR	CIAN
ADAM	MICHAEL
JAMES	JAMIE

AARON	MARK
DYLAN	NATHAN
THOMAS	CIARÁN
RYAN	SAMUEL
DARRAGH	CATHAL
OISÍN	CHARLIE
MATTHEW	ROBERT
JOHN	KYLE
PATRICK	FIONN
BEN	JOSEPH
DAVID	HARRY
CALLUM	CORMAC
ALEX	ANDREW
SHANE	CALUM
EVAN	RORY
EOIN	STEPHEN
JOSHUA	RONAN
CILLIAN	KEVIN
JAKE	NOAH
LIAM	EOGHAN

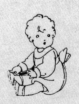

Girls

SARAH	MOLLY
EMMA	ROÍSÍN
KATIE	AISLING
AOIFE	SAOIRSE
SOPHIE	ELLIE
AVA	ABBIE
GRACE	MEGAN
ELLA	HOLLY
LEAH	ELLEN
CLARA	ERIN
AMY	NICOLE
EMILY	ÁINE
LUCY	TARA
CHLOE	SHAUNA
CAOIMHE	CLODAGH
HANNAH	RUBY
RACHEL	LILY
NIAMH	KATELYN
REBECCA	ABIGAIL
JESSICA	EVA
ANNA	CAITLIN
LAUREN	ZOE
KATE	EIMEAR
LAURA	SHANNON
MIA	ISABELLE

And here are the Top Ten in Northern Ireland, reflecting a somewhat more conservative picture:

JACK	KATIE
JAMES	GRACE
MATTHEW	SOPHIE
DANIEL	LUCY
RYAN	EMMA
THOMAS	ELLIE
ADAM	SARAH
JOSHUA	ERIN
DYLAN	HANNAH
BEN	ANNA

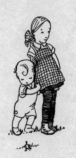

Senan

Going Up

nd which are the names rising fastest up the ladder, those on the cusp of mega-popularity? In the last year counted, there were two first-time entries in the boys' Top 100: Senan and Tristan, while girls' names new to the list were Aoibheann, Aoibhinn and Jasmine. Among other names on the rise:

Girls

ALANA	ELLIE	LUCY
AMELIA	FAYE	MIA
AOIBHE	GRACE	RUBY
AVA	ISABELLA	SARAH
EABHA	ISABELLE	SOPHIE
ELLA	KAYLA	

Boys

CALLUM/Calum	FIONN	OSCAR
CAMERON	LEO	RÍAN
CHARLIE	MAX	RUAIRÍ
CILLIAN	NOAH	SAM
EVAN	OISÍN	

In Northern Ireland, the fastest growing boy's name is Carter, followed by Rory and Aodhán, and for girls Kayleigh, Lucie and Poppy are on the rise. Looking at it locally, in Derry the top names were Callum and Ellie.

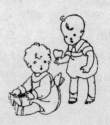

Brady

Irish Exports

For many decades, lively Irish names have been a prime export to the UK and the USA – dating back to the eras of Bridget, Kathleen and Eileen, Kevin, Kelly, Brian, Shannon and Seán. The trend not only continues but has accelerated in both realms.

TOP IRISH NAMES in the UK

Girls

ERIN	NIAMH
CAITLIN	SHANNON
KEIRA	

Boys

RYAN	BRANDON
LIAM	RILEY
CONNOR	AIDAN
FINLAY/Finley	SEAN
KIERAN	

....and

TOP IRISH NAMES in the USA

Girls

RILEY

ERIN

REAGAN

DELANEY

CASSIDY

CAITLIN

KELLY

MCKENNA

SHANNON

CASEY

TEAGAN

RYAN

TARA

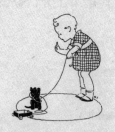

Boys

AIDAN/Aiden	COLIN
RYAN	NOLAN
BRANDON	BRODY
KEVIN	SHAWN
CONNOR	SHANE
SEAN	BRENDAN
BRIAN	DONOVAN
LIAM	KEEGAN
RILEY	QUINN
BRADY	CASEY

COOLEST
EXPORT NAME
• • •
Donovan

Ruairí

Blondes, Brunettes and Especially Redheads

An ever-growing number of parents subscribe to the belief that you shouldn't name a child until you see what he or she looks like. A number of traditional Irish names fit in with this notion, meaning 'fair' or 'dark' or 'red-haired'. The catch, of course, is that a baby's colouring at birth may differ considerably from what it is a year – or ten or twenty – down the road.

Many of the earliest Irish names connote dark colouring or dark hair – perhaps a hint that the Gaels who arrived around the time of Christ came from Spain. Fair colouring was more unusual among the early Irish, and so more prized, with mythical and heavenly creatures often described as having golden hair. The Vikings, who invaded

Ireland in the ninth and tenth centuries, made blonde and red hair more common.

You may want to consider one of these colourful choices for your own little blonde, brunette or redhead.

NAMES for DARK BABIES

Girls

BARRDHUBH

BRENNA

CAREY

CIAR

CIARA/Keara/Kiera/Kira

CIARNAIT

DUIBHEASA/Duvessa

DUIBHLEAMHNA

DÚINSEACH

KERRY

ORNA

Boys

BRANDUBH/Branduff

CIARAN/Kieran

CIARMHAC

CRÓNÁN/Cronan

DOLAN

DONNCHADH/Donagh

DONAHUE

DONLEAVY

DONN

DONNABHÁN/Donovan

DONNAGÁN/Donegan

DONNÁN

DOUGAL

DOYLE

DUALTACH/Duald

DUBHÁN/Duane

DUBH/Duff

DUBHAGÁN/Duggan

DUBHDARA

FEARDORCHA/Farry

KERWIN

SULLIVAN

TEIMHNÍN/Tynan

Either

DARCY

DELANEY

DONNELLY

DUBHÓG

DUBHTHACH/Dufach

DUFFY

GORMAN

NAMES for FAIR BABIES

Girls

BÁINE

BÉIBHINN/Bevin

CAOILINN/Keelin

CAOIMHINN

CEALLACH/Kelly

CÉIBHIONN

FINNEACHT

FINNÉADAN

FINNSEACH

FIONA

FIONNUALA/Finola

FIONNÚIR

MUIREANN

MUIRGHEAL/Muriel

NIAMH

NUALA

UAINIONN

Boys

CAOIMHÍN/Kevin

FINN

FINNBARR

FINNEGAN

FINNIAN

FINTAN

LACHTNA

ORAN

Either

AILBHE/Alby

ALBANY

BAIRRFHIONN/Barry

MOINGIONN

NAMES for RED-HAIRED BABIES

Girls

COCHRANN

CORCAIR

FLANNAIT

RÓISÍN

SCARLETT

Boys

ALROY

CORC

CORCRÁN/Corcoran

DEARGÁN

FLANNÁN

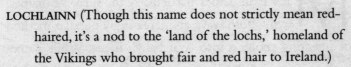

LOCHLAINN (Though this name does not strictly mean red-haired, it's a nod to the 'land of the lochs,' homeland of the Vikings who brought fair and red hair to Ireland.)

REED/Reid

ROAN/Rohan

ROONE/Rooney

Either

CLANCY

DERRY

FLANN

FLANAGAN

FLANNERY

FLYNN

RUAIRÍ/Rory

ROWAN

Darragh

Irish Unisex Names

Many Irish names, particularly the surname-names, swing both ways, an increasingly popular method of injecting coolness into your baby's name. While names such as Kerry and Kelly, once used for boys as well as girls, have largely shifted to the female side, a whole new raft of choices has arrived to take their place. Here is a selection of names equally appropriate, not to mention cool, for both girls and boys.

AILBHE	CASSIDY
ALBANY	CHRISTIAN
BEVIN	CLANCY
CAMPBELL	DARA
CASEY	DARCY

DARRAGH	OWNY
DELANEY	QUINN
DERRY	REAGAN/Regan
DONNELLY	RILEY
DUFFY	RORY
EVANY	ROWAN
FALLON	RYAN
FARRELL	SHEA
FLANN	TIERNAN
FLANAGAN	TIERNEY
FLANNERY	
FLYNN	
GORMAN	
KENNEDY	
LOGAN	
MAGEE	
MAOLÍOSA	
MORGAN	
MURPHY	

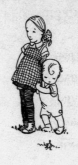

Isla

Pan-Celtic Cool

As Celtic languages have several different branches, you may want to look beyond Irish names to those of your fellow Celts: the Scottish, Welsh, Cornish, Breton and even the Manx, from the Isle of Man. As with Irish names, many of these are being revived in their native lands, offering the perfect blend of tradition and exotic cool. Note that a few of the boys' names – Dylan, Idris, Reese – would work and perhaps be even cooler for girls.

Girls

AALIN	Manx
AAMOR	Breton
ADARYN	Welsh
ADIGIS	Cornish

ADO	Cornish
AELA	Breton
AELWEN	Welsh
AERONA	Welsh
AFTON	Scottish
AILSA	Scottish
AINSLEY	Scottish
ALIENOR	Breton
ALMEDA	Breton
ANCHORET	Welsh
ANEIRA	Welsh
ANGHARAD	Welsh
ARWEN	Welsh
AZENOR	Breton
BERIANA	Cornish
BLODWEN	Welsh
BRANWEN	Welsh
BRONWEN	Welsh
BRYN/BRYNNA	Welsh
BRYONY	Welsh
CERIDWEN	Welsh
CERYS	Welsh
CORALIE	Breton
DELWEN	Welsh
DEMELZA	Cornish
DERRYTH	Welsh
DWYN	Welsh
EILWEN	Welsh

ELSPETH	Scottish
ELUNED	Welsh
ENDELIENT	Cornish
ENORA	Breton
ERTHA	Cornish
ERWANEZ	Breton
FFION	Welsh
GAYNOR	Welsh
GETHAN	Welsh
GLENYS/Glynis	Welsh
GWANWEN	Welsh
GWEN/Wenn	Cornish
GWYNETH	Welsh
HAUDE	Breton
IA	Cornish
IGERNA	Cornish
INEDA	Cornish
INIRA	Welsh
IONA/Ione	Scottish
ISLA	Scottish
IVORI	Welsh
KATELL	Breton
KERENZA	Cornish
KEW	Cornish
KEYNE	Cornish
MABAN	Welsh
MADRUN	Cornish
MAILLI	Cornish

MEDWENNA	Welsh
MELLE	Breton
MEREWIN	Cornish
MINIVER	Cornish
MORAG	Scottish
MWYNEN	Welsh
MYFANWY	Welsh
NERYS	Welsh
NEVID(D)	Cornish, Welsh
NEWLYN	Welsh
NONN/Nonna	Cornish
OANEZ	Breton
OLWEN	Welsh
PIALA	Cornish, Breton
RHEDYN	Welsh
RHIAN/Rhiannon	Welsh
RHIANWEN	Welsh
RHONWEN	Welsh
ROZENN	Breton
SCÁTHACH	Scottish
SEIRIAN	Welsh
SERERENA	Cornish
SEVE/SEVA	Breton
SIAN	Welsh
TAMSIN	Cornish
TEGWEN	Welsh
WENN(A)	Cornish
WYNN(E)	Welsh

Boys

ACCALON	Breton
ADEON	Welsh
AEL	Breton
ANGUS	Scottish
ALASDAIR	Scottish
ALED	Welsh
ALEF	Cornish
AMATHEON	Welsh
ANARAWD	Welsh
ANEURIN	Welsh
ANGWYN	Welsh
ANNAN	Scottish
ARDAN	Scottish
ARGYLE	Scottish
ATHOL	Scottish
AURON	Welsh
AUSTELL	Cornish
BANADEL	Welsh
BAIRD	Scottish
BASTIAN	Breton
BERWIN	Cornish
BLAZEY	Cornish
BOWEN	Welsh
BRANWELL	Cornish
BRASTIUS	Cornish
BRECON	Welsh

BREIZH	Breton
BRICE/Bryce	Welsh
BRYN	Welsh
BUCHANAN	Scottish
CADOC	Welsh
CAMBER	Welsh
CANNOCK/ Kinnock	Cornish
CARADOC	Welsh
CARANTEC	Breton
CASWALLAWN	Welsh
CLEDWIN	Welsh
CORENTIN(E)	Breton
DAWE	Welsh
DENZEL(L)	Cornish
DOCCO	Cornish
DRYSTAN	Welsh
DUGALD	Scottish
DUNCAN	Scottish
DYLAN	Welsh
EDERN	Cornish
EDRYD	Welsh
EIROS	Welsh
ELFED	Welsh
ELPHIN	Welsh
EMLYN	Welsh
EMRYS	Welsh
EWAN/Ewen	Scottish
EVAN	Welsh

FARQUAR	Scottish
FERGUS/Ferguson	Scottish
FIFE/Fyfe	Scottish
FORBES	Scottish
FRASER/Frazier	Scottish
GAIR	Scottish
GARETH	Welsh
GAWAIN	Cornish, Welsh
GERWYN	Welsh
GLYN	Welsh
GRAHAM	Scottish
GREGOR	Scottish
GRIFFITH	Welsh
GUTHRIE	Scottish
GWYNFOR	Welsh
HACO	Cornish
HAMISH	Scottish
HYWEL	Welsh
IDRIS	Welsh
IDWAL	Welsh
IFOR	Welsh
INIR/Ynyr	Welsh
INNIS	Scottish
JAGO	Cornish
JOB/Jos	Breton
KEIR	Scottish
KELVIN	Scottish
KENDRICK	Scottish

KENTIGERN	Breton
KYLE	Scottish
KYNON	Welsh, Cornish
LENNOX	Scottish
LLEWELLYN	Welsh
MADOC/Madeg	Breton
MALCOLM	Scottish
MATH	Welsh
MAXEN	Welsh
MELAN	Cornish, Breton
MELOR	Breton
MORAY	Scottish
MUNGO	Scottish
NYE	Welsh
OGILVY	Scottish
ONILWYN	Welsh
PENWYN	Welsh
PETROC	Cornish
RAMSEY	Manx
RHYS/Reese	Welsh
RHAIN	Welsh
RHYDACH/Riddock	Cornish
RHYDWYN	Welsh
RUMO/Rumon	Cornish
SENAN	Cornish
STRACHAN	Scottish
SULIAN/Sulien	Breton, Welsh
TALIESIN	Welsh

TANGUY/Tangi	Breton
TORIN	Cornish, Manx
TOSTIG	Welsh
TREMAINE/Tremayne	Cornish
TREVELYAN	Cornish
URIEN	Welsh, Breton
URQUHART	Scottish
VAUGHAN	Welsh
VISANT	Breton
WYNFORD	Welsh
WYNN	Welsh
YESTIN	Welsh

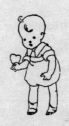

Cadence

Non-Irish Cool

Ireland and the Irish may be cooler than anyplace or anyone, but let's face it: French clothes, Italian shoes, German art, American music, Russian supermodels – there's cool beyond our shores, too. In case you want to investigate cool *non*-Irish names for your baby, here are some choices currently in vogue throughout Europe and in the USA.

Girls

ADDISON	
ALESSIA	FLAVIE
ALLEGRA	FLORA
CADENCE	FRANCESCA
CLAUDIA	GAIA
COSIMA	GIANNA
DANICA	GINEVRA
ELIANA	ILARIA
FEDERICA	INÈS

IRIS

ISABELLA

JADA

LÉA

LENA

LETICIA

LILA

LOLA

LUCIA

LUDOVICA

LUNA

MANON

MARINE

NATALYA

NEVAEH (heaven spelled
backwards)

OCÉANE

PALOMA

PETRA

POPPY

ROMY

RUBY

SADIE

SANNE

SOPHIE

TATIANA

VIOLA

Boys

ALEXEI

ANDREAS

CADEN

CLEMENS

COLE

DANE

ELIAS

ENZO

FABIAN

FELIX

FILIPPO

HUDSON

ISAAC

IVAN

KRISTOF

LORENZO

MAGNUS

MARCOS

MATEO

MAXIMILIAN

MILLER

NICO

SEM

STONE

TANCREDI

THEO

TIBOR

WOLF

WYATT

Either

ADRIAN

DAKOTA

JUSTICE

LUCA

MILAN

PEYTON

PRESLEY

SASHA

SAWYER

TRUE

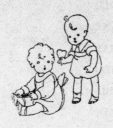

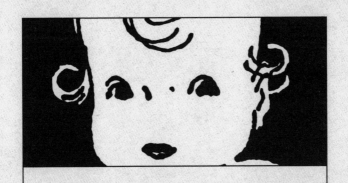

II. COOL COOL

...

Famous Names

Cillian

Cool Irish Celeb Names

There's no question that being attached to a celebrity – of the past or of the present – sprinkles a certain stardust on a name, and in this celebrity-driven culture this has become a more and more influential element in baby naming. Some celebrity names are inspiring thousands of namesakes across various cultures – the glamorous Ava, for example, is now seen on popularity lists from Scotland to Scandinavia.

The following lists include inspirational Irish-named celebrities, mostly drawn from the worlds of entertainment and literature:

AIDAN QUINN

AISLING O'SULLIVAN

ARDAL O'HANLON

BONO (b. Paul Hewson)

BRID BRENNAN

BRONAGH GALLAGHER

CATHAL COUGHLAN

CIARÁN HINDS

CILLIAN MURPHY

CLODAGH ROGERS

COLIN FARRELL

COLM MEANEY

CONAN O'BRIEN

COLUM McCANN

CORMAC McCARTHY

DAIRE BREHAN

DARAGH O'MALLEY

DERVLA KIRWAN

DEVON MICHAEL MURRAY

EAMONN CAMPBELL (The Dubliners)

EAVAN AISLING BOLAND

ELVIS (b. Declan) COSTELLO

EMER MARTIN

ENYA (b. Eithne)

EOIN COLFER

FEARGAL LAWLER (The Cranberries)

FEARGAL (b. Sean) SHARKEY

FERDIA MACANNA

FINTAN MCKEOWN

FIONA SHAW

FIONNULA FLANAGAN

GAY (b. Gabriel, nickname Gaybo) BYRNE

LAOISE KELLY

LIAM NEESON

MAEVE BINCHY

MÁIRE NÍ BHRAOÁIN

MALACHI CUSH

MALACHY McCOURT

MILO O'SHEA

NIALL TOIBIN

NIAMH CUSACK

NOLAN RYAN

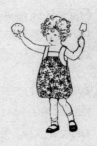

ORLA FITZGERALD

PADDY CASEY

PÁDRAIC BREATHNACH

PÁDRAIC DELANEY

PHELIM DREW

PIERCE BROSNAN

REDMOND O'HANLON

RODEN NOEL

RÓISÍN MURPHY

ROMA DOWNEY

RORY GALLAGHER

RÚAIDHRI CONROY

SAOIRSE RONAN

SEAMUS HEANEY

SINÉAD O'CONNOR

SIOBHAN MCCARTHY

SLAINE KELLY

SORCHA CUSACK

VAN MORRISON

COOLEST
CELEB NAME
...
Saoirse

Rafferty

Starbabies with Irish Names

Celebrities on both sides of the Atlantic, those with and without Hibernian roots, have long been partial to Irish names. Here are some of the coolest, along with our reasons for thinking so:

AIDAN *Scott Hamilton (Olympic figure skater), Robert F Kennedy, Jr*
Once a pet form of Aodh, which means 'little fire', Aidan is spreading like wildfire from Edinburgh to Pittsburgh, prized for its strength and charm. Also seen as Aédán, Aodhán, Aiden, Eadan and Edan (not to mention Aidyn, Ayden, Adon and countless other 'creative forms').

AOIFE *Ciarán Hinds*
Popular name dating back to a fierce woman warrior in early myth, it has been anglicised as Eva and Ava.

BECKETT *Malcolm McDowell, Melissa Etheridge*

An appealing last-name name rich in literary associations, both to the play and film based on the life of St Thomas à B. and to the Irish playwright-novelist Samuel B., it's red hot in Hollywood.

BRIAN *Nancy Kerrigan*

The skating champ went with this perennial, tried-and-true favourite, the namesake of Brian Boru, legendary Irish warrior-king.

CASHEL *Daniel Day-Lewis*

The Irish actor and his American wife chose an unusual Irish place name for their son; it's also seen as Caisel.

CIARÁN *Padraig Harrington*

The internationally known champion golfer chose a name that's growing in popularity, in both this and in the Kieran spelling that was used by actress Julianna Margulies.

COLIN *Paul Stanley*

The member of iconic ghoul rock group Kiss picked this perennially popular offshoot of Nicholas.

CONNOR *Nicole Kidman and Tom Cruise*

Spelled with one *n* or two, this anglicised version of

Conchobhar, renowned in Irish myth, has long been popular in Eire and is climbing the popularity lists of other countries as well.

DARBY *Patrick Dempsey*
Disney's *Darby O'Gill and the Little People* made this spirited, light-hearted name seem more Irish than it actually is.

DONOVAN *Charisma Carpenter (of Buffy, the Vampire Slayer fame), Noel Gallagher*
Another appealing last-name name, this one has long outgrown its 'Mellow Yellow' associations.

EVER *Milla Jovovich and Paul Anderson*
In addition to being an evocative word name, this is an Anglicisation of the Irish Éibhear, originating with one of the mythic leaders of the first Gaelic settlers in Ireland.

FINLEY *Chris O'Donnell*
One of the newly popular Fin-family of names, also spelled Finlay (as used by Sadie Frost).

FINN *Christy Turlington and Ed Burns, Jane Leeves, Andrea Catherwood*
This is a name with enormous energy and charm, that of the greatest hero of Irish myth, Finn MacCool. Other

related cool starbaby names: FLYNN (Elle Macpherson), and FINNIGAN (Eric McCormack of *Will & Grace* fame), not to mention Julia Roberts' phabulous Phinnaeus.

FIONA *Jenny Garth*
Although this name is a Scottish invention, it has an Irish feel and is commonly found among the Finolas and Fion-nualas.

GULLIVER *Gary Oldman, Damian Lewis*
This relatively rare Gaelic surname was known primarily through his literary *Travels* until actor Oldman transformed it into a lively baby-name option.

HONOR *Tilda Swinton*
Though not Celtic in origin, this upstanding virtue name has long been used in Ireland, along with others like Grace and Faith.

IRELAND *Kim Basinger and Alec Baldwin*
If Ireland isn't Irish, what is?

JAMES PADRAIG *Colin Farrell*
Cool combination of classic New Testament name with one of the many versions of the name of Ireland's patron saint.

KIAN *Geena Davis*

This spelling variation of Cian was chosen by the actress for one of her twin boys. The other twin's name is Kaiis.

LENNON *Patsy Kensit and Liam Gallagher*

Naming a child after your cultural or other hero gives him two cool advantages: a name with real meaning and a positive image to reach towards. Another rocker, Zakk Wylde, chose Hendrix as his son's musical hero name.

LIAM *Calista Flockhart, Tori Spelling*

Sprightly and richly textured classic that started as a short form of William.

MAEVE *Chris O'Donnell*

An early Irish goddess and queen name, short but strong, now catching on across the pond. The O'Donnells named another of their five children Finley.

MALACHY *Cillian Murphy*

An Irish version of a biblical name, with an expansive, almost boisterous image.

MICHEAL *Liam Neeson and Natasha Richardson*

The Northern Irish star stuck to the Gaelic spelling of the enduring Michael for his first son.

MILO *Ricki Lake, Liz Tyler, Sherry Springfield (of* ER *fame)*
Jaunty Irish spin on Miles.

OSCAR *Gillian Anderson, Hugh Jackman*
This amiable Victorian favourite is having a definite revival among stylish parents on both sides of the Atlantic.

PADDY *Mare Winningham*
One of the most enduring nickname names.

QUINLIN *Ben Stiller*
A strong surname name usually spelled Quinlan that could make a child feel distinctive while still having the easy-to-handle nickname of Quinn.

QUINN *Sharon Stone*
'The mighty Quinn' is a unisex name that's strong for both genders.

RAFFERTY *Sadie Frost and Jude Law*
One of the coolest of the Irish surnames, with a raffish quality all its own.

REILLY *Roma Downey*
There are Reillys and Rileys galore crossing both continental and gender lines.

RHIANNON *Robert Rodriguez*

The combination makes for an appealing cross-cultural mix. Some might consider it an improvement over the names of the 'Spy Kids' director's four sons: Rebel, Rocket, Racer and Rogue.

RILEY *David Lynch*
See *Reilly.*

ROAN *Sharon Stone*
A strong, red-haired choice.

RÓISÍN *Sinéad O'Connor*
An authentic selection for a little Irish rose.

RONAN *Rebecca Miller and Daniel Day-Lewis*
Compelling, legendary name of ten Celtic saints.

ROWAN *Brooke Shields*
This friendly Irish last name was almost unheard of as a girl's name before Brooke Shields made the gender switch; now it shows lots of potential as a likeable, unisex choice.

RYAN *Pete Sampras*
Classic.

SULLIVAN   *Patrick Dempsey*

A jaunty Irish surname name with a real twinkle in its eye, used for the twin of Darby.

TALLULAH   *Patrick Dempsey, Simon LeBon, Demi Moore and Bruce Willis*

The then Willises almost single-handedly launched the cool starbaby name concept when they chose Scout and Rumer as well as the more user-friendly Tallulah for their girls. This anglicisation of Tuilelaith is now being picked up on by other celeb parents.

…And some other names chosen by Irish and Irish-American notables:

BONO   *Jordan, Memphis Eve, John Abraham, Elijah Bob Patricus, Guggi Q*

PIERCE BROSNAN   *Seán, Dylan Thomas, Paris Beckett*

ED BURNS   *Grace (and Finn)*

GABRIEL BYRNE   *Jack Daniel, Romy Marion*

DAVE (THE EDGE) EVANS   *Hollie, Arun, Blue Angel, Sian*

LIAM GALLAGHER   *Gene, Molly (and Lennon)*

NOEL GALLAGHER   *Rory, Anais (and Donovan)*

DENIS LEARY   *Jack, Devin*

DAMIEN LEITH   *Jagger Ramone*

EDELE LYNCH   *Ceol Sheila*

ORLAITH MCALLISTER   *Eva*

JOEY MCINTYRE   *Griffin Thomas*

LIAM NEESON   *Daniel Jack (and Micheal)*

SINÉAD O'CONNOR   *Jake, Shane, Yeshua (and Róisín)*

DOLORES O'RIORDAN   *Taylor Baxter, Molly, Dakota Rain*

PETER O'TOOLE   *Kate, Patricia, Lorcan*

AIDAN QUINN   *Ava Eileen*

STEPHEN REA   *Danny, Oscar*

Artemis

Characters from Irish Literature

Here, some literary inspiration suggestions coming from characters found in the pages of books spanning various periods of literary history. But in this category, as always, feel free to think about your own personal favourites.

Female

CHARACTER	AUTHOR	BOOK
ADA	Anne Enright	*The Gathering*
AISLING	Maeve Binchy	*Light a Penny Candle*
AROON	Molly Keane	*Good Behaviour*
BABA (Bridget)	Edna O'Brien	*The Country Girls*
BRIDIE	William Trevor	*The Ballroom of Romance*
CAITHLEEN	Edna O'Brien	*The Country Girls*

CHARACTER	AUTHOR	BOOK
CARMILLA	Sheridan Le Fanu	*Carmilla*
CATALINA	Edna O'Brien	*The High Road*
CIARA	Colum McCann	*A Word in Edgewise*
EIBHLÍN	Mícheál O'Guiheen	*A Pity Youth Does Not Last*
ELLENA	Richard Brinsley Sheridan	*The Critic*
EVERGREEN	Brian Cleeve	*Judith*
HONOR	Iris Murdoch	*A Severed Head*
IMELDA	Roddy Doyle	*The Commitments*
IMOGEN	Aidan Higgins	*Langrishe Go Down*
ISOLT	Emer Martin	*Breakfast in Babylon*
ITA	Anne Enright	*The Gathering*
FIANNA	Edna O'Brien	*The Heather Blazing*
KAHEENA	Eoin Colfer	*Benny & Omar*
LETTY	William Trevor	*Reading Turgenev*
MARDA	Elizabeth Bowen	*The Last September*
MAURYA	Jennifer Johnston	*Old Jest*
MELODY	Roddy Doyle	*A Star Called Henry*
MINNIE	Christopher Nolan	*The Banyan Tree*
MOIRA	Colum McCann	*A Word in Edgewise*
NUALA	Christopher Nolan	*The Banyan Tree*
ORNA	Eoin Colfer	*Benny & Omar*
PEIG	Maurice O'Sullivan★	*Twenty Years a' Growing*
RAIN	Iris Murdoch	*The Sandcastle*
SAOIRSE	Cecilia Ahern	*If You Could See Me Now*
TALLIS	Iris Murdoch	*A Fairly Honourable Defeat*

★*also known as Muiris Ó Súilleabháin*

Male

CHARACTER	AUTHOR	BOOK
ARTEMIS	Eoin Colfer	*Artemis Fowl* series
BALTHAZAR	J P Donleavy	*The Beastly Beatitudes of Balthazar B.*
BEC	Darren Shan	*Bec*
CATO	Iris Murdoch	*Henry and Cato*
CHARLO	Roddy Doyle	*The Woman Who Walked Into Doors*
DANBY	Iris Murdoch	*Bruno's Dream*
DECLAN	Colm Toíbín	*The Blackwater Lightship*
DECO	Roddy Doyle	*The Commitments*
DEKKO	William Trevor	*Beyond the Pale*
DORIAN	Oscar Wilde	*The Picture of Dorian Gray*
DOYLER	Jamie O'Neill	*At Swim, Two Boys*
EAMON	Edna O'Brien	*The Heather Blazing*
EOIN	Colum McCann	*A Word in Edgewise*
ENDA	Julia O'Faolain	*A Pot of Soothing Herbs*
GYPO	Liam O'Flaherty	*The Informer*
HUGO	Iris Murdoch	*Under the Net*
IVOR	Anne Enright	*The Gathering*
JEM	Anne Enright	*The Gathering*
KIERAN	Colum McCann	*A Word in Edgewise*
LORCAN	Eoin Colfer	*Benny & Omar*
MALACHY	Patrick McCabe	*The Dead School*
MICKAH	Roddy Doyle	*The Commitments*

CHARACTER	AUTHOR	BOOK
MOR	Iris Murdoch	*The Sandcastle*
MOSS	Anne Enright	*The Gathering*
MUIRIS	Michéal O'Guiheen	*A Pity Youth Does Not Last*
MYLES	John Banville	*The Sea*
NIALL	Eoin Colfer	*Benny & Omar*
PÁDRAIG	Micheál O'Guiheen	*A Pity Youth Does Not Last*
PHELIM	Thomas Keneally	*Bring Larks and Heroes*
QUINTY	William Trevor	*My House in Umbria*
RONAN	Eoin Colfer	*Benny & Omar*
SEAGRUN	Brian Cleeve	*Tread Softly in This Place*
SEBASTIAN	J P Donleavy	*The Ginger Man*
SWEENEY	Flann O'Brien	*At Swim-Two-Birds*
TALLIS	Iris Murdoch	*A Fairly Honourable Defeat*
TARRY	Patric Kavanagh	*Tarry Flynn*
TOMÁS	Maurice O'Sullivan★	*Twenty Years a' Growing*
VIRGILIUS	Sean O'Faolain	*The Man Who Invented Sin*

★*also known as Muiris Ó Súilleabháin*

Xenia

Names from James Joyce

It's not easy to pluck names from the works of a writer who calls characters Gush and Roaring, Mutt and Butt. They range from the reasonably straightforward in *The Dubliners* to the somewhat riskier in *Ulysses* to the every-man-for-himself in *Finnegan's Wake*. Here are some of the more user friendly.

Female

ADA	ELIZA
ANNA LIVIA	EVELINE
ANNIE	GILLIA
BEATRICE	IRIS
CELIA	JULIA
DELIA	KATE

KATHLEEN	OLIVE
KITTY	PHILOMENA
LILI	PHOEBE
LILY	POLLY
LISA	UNA
MARIA	WINNIE
MINA	XENIA
MOLLY	
MORNA	

Male

ALEXANDER
ANDREW
BANTAM
BARNEY
BARTELL
BLAZES
BRIAN
CLIVE
CONOLLY
DENIS
DUNBAR
FINN
GABRIEL
GARRETT
HUGH

**JAMES JOYCE'S
ABC's**

• • •

There's Ada, Bett, Celia, Delia, Ena, Fretta, Gilda, Hilda, Itra, Jess, Katty, Lou (they make me cough as sure as I read them), Mina, Nippa, Opsy, Poll, Queeniee, Ruth, Saucy, Trix, Una, Vela, Wanda, Xenia, Yva, Zulma, Phoebe, Thelma. And Mee!

—*Finnegan's Wake*

IGNATIUS

KEVIN

LANTY

LEO

LEOPOLD

MALACHI

MYLES

NATHAN

NED

O'CONNOR

PATRICK/Paddy/Patsy

REUBEN

ROCHE

SEÁN/Shaun

SHEMUS

SIMON

SMITH

STEPHEN

TERENCE/Terry

VALENTINE

WISDOM

GARDEN OF NAMES

• • •

Winnie, Olive and Beatrice, Nelly and Ida, Amy and Rue. Here they come, all the gay pack, for they are the florals, from foncey and pansey to papavere's blush, foresake-me-nought, while there's leaf there's hope, with primtim's ruse and marrymay's blossom, all the flowers of the ancelles' garden.

—Finnegan's Wake

Juno

Stage Names

Here, a menu of evocative names from the plays of four of Ireland's greatest playwrights, William Butler Yeats, George Bernard Shaw, Sean O'Casey and J M Synge:

Female

NAME	PLAYWRIGHT	PLAY
AMARYLLIS	Shaw	*Back to Methuselah*
ARIADNE	Shaw	*Heartbreak House*
BRIDGET	Yeats	*The Land of Heart's Desire*
CANDIDA	Shaw	*Candida*
CATHLEEN	Yeats	*The Countess Cathleen*
	Synge	*Riders to the Sea*
CHLOE	Shaw	*Back to Methuselah*
DECIMA	Yeats	*The Player Queen*

NAME	PLAYWRIGHT	PLAY
DEIRDRE	Yeats	*Deirdre*
	Synge	*Deirdre of the Sorrows*
DELIA	Yeats	*Cathleen ni Houlihan*
EEADA	O'Casey	*Red Roses for Me*
ELIZA	Shaw	*Pygmalion*
EPIFANIA	Shaw	*The Millionairess*
FINNOOLA	O'Casey	*Red Roses for Me*
HONOR	Synge	*The Playboy of the Western World*
HYPATIA	Shaw	*Misalliance*
JUNO	O'Casey	*Juno and the Paycock*
LAVARCHAM	Synge	*Deirdre of the Sorrows*
LILITH	Shaw	*Back to Methuselah*
MAISIE	O'Casey	*Juno and the Paycock*
MAURTEEN	Yeats	*The Land of Heart's Desire*
MAURYA	Synge	*Riders to the Sea*
MINNIE	O'Casey	*The Shadow of a Gunman*
MOLLY	Synge	*The Well of the Saints*
NONA	Yeats	*The Player Queen*
NORA	O'Casey	*The Plough and the Stars*
	Synge	*Riders to the Sea*
OONA	Yeats	*The Countess Cathleen*
ORINTHIA	Shaw	*The Apple Cart*
PEGEEN	Synge	*The Playboy of the Western World*
PAUDEEN	Yeats	*The Unicorn from the Stars*
RAINA	Shaw	*Arms and the Man*
SIBBY	Yeats	*The Pot of Broth*
SOUHAIN	O'Casey	*Purple Dust*

Male

NAME	PLAYWRIGHT	PLAY
ADOLPHUS	Shaw	*Major Barbara*
AINNLE	Synge	*Deirdre of the Sorrows*
ALEEL	Yeats	*The Countess Cathleen*
ARDAN	Synge	*Deirdre of the Sorrows*
AYAMONN	O'Casey	*Red Roses for Me*
BARTLEY	Synge	*Riders to the Sea*
CASHEL	Shaw	*The Admirable Bashville*
COLENSO	Shaw	*The Doctor's Dilemma*
CONCHUBOR	Synge	*Deirdre of the Sorrows*
CUTLER	Shaw	*The Doctor's Dilemma*
EMER	Yeats	*The Only Jealousy of Emer*
FERGIS	Synge	*Deirdre of the Sorrows*
FERGUS	Yeats	*Deirdre*
	Shaw	*You Never Can Tell*
FINCH	Shaw	*You Never Can Tell*
MAGNUS	Shaw	*Androcles and the Lion*
NAISI	Synge	*Deirdre of the Sorrow*
NAOISE	Yeats	*Deirdre*
OCTAVIUS	Shaw	*Man and Superman*
OWEN	Synge	*Deirdre of the Sorrows*
PATRICK	Yeats	*Cathleen ni Houlihan*
ROORY	O'Casey	*Red Roses for Me*
SERGIUS	Shaw	*Arms and the Man*
SEUMAS	O'Casey	*The Shadow of a Gunman*

NAME	PLAYWRIGHT	PLAY
SHAWN	Synge	*The Playboy of the Western World*
	Yeats	*The Land of Heart's Desire*
SHEMUS	Yeats	*The Countess Cathleen*
TEIGUE	Yeats	*The Countess Cathleen*
VALENTINE	Shaw	*You Never Can Tell*
ZOZIM	Shaw	*Back to Methuselah*

COOLEST
STAGE NAME
• • •
Juno

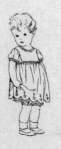

Sholeh

Seen On Screen

Name inspiration can come from almost anywhere, including your TV and film screens. Here, first, are some examples of characters that have appeared on the video screen, from popular soap operas to sitcoms to more serious fare:

ALI	*Fair City*
AOIRGHE	*Eureka Street*
CLEO	*Fair City*
COLUM	*Scarlett*
DOUGAL	*Father Ted*
EILISH	*Single-Handed*
EITHNE	*Seacht*

FINBARR	*Single-Handed*
KYLIE	*Fair City*
LOÏC	*Dolmen*
LORCAN	*Fair City*
MAGS	*Fair City*
MALACHY	*Fair City*
MONDO	*Fair City*
NIAMH	*Fair City*
PASCAL	*Fair City*
RORY	*Pride and Joy*
SEAMUS	*Fair City*
SHOLEH	*Fair City*

And from the big screen:

BERNADETTE	*The Wind That Shakes the Barley*
CARMEL	*Pete's Meteor*
CHRISTY (male)	*My Left Foot*
COCO	*Strength and Honour*
CON	*Rory O'Shea Was Here*
CONNOR	*Road to Perdition*
CONZO	*Goldfish Memory*
CRISPINA	*The Magdalene Sisters*

DAMIEN	*The Wind That Shakes the Barley*
DEIRDRE	*Intermission*
DERMOT	*Agnes Browne*
DONAL	*Conspiracy of Silence*
DYMPNA	*About Adam*
DUNCAN	*Con Air*
EAMON	*The Secret of Roan Inish*
FERGUS	*The Craic*
FINBAR	*The Brothers McMullen*
FINN	*Road to Perdition*
FIONA	*The Secret of Roan Inish*
FLYNN	*The Secret of Roan Inish*
GARETH (female)	*In the Name of the Father*
GEMMA	*Cowboys and Angels*
HUBIE	*Tara Road*
ISOLDE	*Goldfish Memory*
JIMEOIN	*The Craic*
LIAM	*Michael Collins*
LEHIFF	*Intermission*
MAISIE	*The Boys and Girls from County Clare*
MAJELLA	*Conspiracy of Silence*
MICHEAIL	*The Wind That Shakes the Barley*
MIKO	*The Boys and Girls from County Clare*
MO CHARA	*Man About Dog*

NOELEEN	*Intermission*
NIALL	*When Brendan Met Trudy*
NUALA	*When Brendan Met Trudy*
PHELIM	*Rat*
RORY	*Rory O'Shea Was Here*
SADIE	*My Left Foot*
SCUD	*Man About Dog*
SHAMUS	*Puckoon*
SINÉAD	*The Wind That Shakes the Barley*
SIOBHAN	*Rory O'Shea Was Here*
TADGH	*The Field; The Secret of Roan Inish*
WHEELER	*Strength and Honour*

COOLEST
SCREEN NAME
• • •

*Gareth
for a girl*

Orinthia

Poetic Licence

Writers everywhere sometimes feel constricted by the database of established names and feel moved to invent their own. Irish writers are no exception. The Northern Irish writer C S Lewis was perhaps the most inventive with names in his *Chronicles of Narnia,* which include the males Caspian, Rilian, Shasta and Tirian. More often, however, writers concentrate their naming efforts on female characters. Here is a selection of girls' names that were the inspirations of Irish authors:

ANNA LIVIA
James Joyce drew this name from the ancient Irish name for the river Liffey: Abhainn na Life.

ARAVIS
An invention from C S Lewis's *Chronicles of Narnia.*

DAIREEN

Invented by Limerick author F Frankfort Moore for the title character of his 1893 novel.

GLORIA

Conceived by George Bernard Shaw for the 1898 play *You Never Can Tell*.

GLORVINA

Invented name for a prince's daughter in Lady Morgan's *The Wild Irish Girl*, 1806.

MALVINA

In James Macpherson's Ossianic poems, Malvina was the invented name for the lover of Oscar, grandson of Finn Mac-Cool.

MAURYA

A character in J M Synge's 1904 drama, *Riders to the Sea*.

ORINTHIA

George Bernard Shaw created this name for his 1929 play, *The Apple Cart*.

VEVINA

Form of Béibhinn used in Ossianic poems.

ZAIRA

Invented by the Irish writer C R Maturin for his novel, *Women; or pour et contre*, 1818.

Oisín

Irish Athletes

Many of the legendary stars of sports history tend to have ordinary guy names such as Jack and Jim, Mike and Mick, but the Christian names of some of the more modern stars, as well as some of their last names, offer options that go beyond the perimeters of that limited playing field. Consider these names of Irish sports heroes for your own cool little athlete.

Female

CIARA Grant – football

EMMA Byrne – football

FIONNUALA Britton – track

OLIVE Loughnane – track

OLIVIA O'Toole – football

RÓISÍN McGettigan – track

AINE O'Gorman – football

NIAMH Fahey – football

SONIA O'Sullivan – track

Male

AIDAN O'Keeffe – football

ARMSTRONG Gerry – football

CATHAL Muckian – football

CHRISTY Ring – hurling

CIAN Byrne – football

CIARAIN Fitzgerald – rugby

COLM Cooper – Gaelic football

CONN McCall – cricket

DAMIEN Fitzhenry – hurling

DARRAGH Ó Sé – Gaelic football

DECLAN O'Brien – football

DONAL Óg Cusack – hurling

DUSTY Flanagan – football

ÉAMON Zayed – football

EOIN Kelly – hurling

GEORGE Best – football

HENRY Shefflin – hurling

ISAAC Boss – rugby

JACK Doyle – boxer

KIERAN Donaghy – basketball

LUKE Fitzgerald – rugby

MAIK Taylor – football

MAL Donaghy – football

MARC Ó Sé – Gaelic football

OISÍN McConville – Gaelic football

PADRAIG Harrington – golfer

RAY McLoughlin – rugby

RONAN Curran – hurling

ROY Keane – football

RUBY Walsh – horse-racing

SEÁN Kelly – cycling

SHAY Given – football

STEPHEN Ireland – football

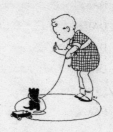

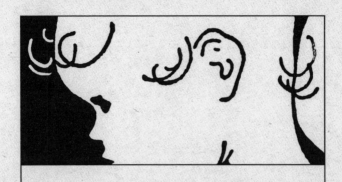

III. PRE-COOL
COOL

...

Old Names

Emer

Names from Irish Myth and Legend

I reland is rich in folk tales and legends starring characters that range from pagan gods and goddesses to ancient kings and queens to the fairies who live in the roots of old trees. But perhaps the greatest Irish legends of them all centre on the mythical hero Finn MacCool, son of a slain warrior and a king's daughter. Raised in secret by a druidess and tutored by a druid, he grows up to become a great warrior with mystical powers derived from sucking his burnt thumb when cooking the Salmon of Knowledge. With the gift of prophecy, Finn uses his magic to save the king and gain command of the military elite. He instills a code of honour and these champions become the followers of Finn, the first Fenians, or Fianna, of Ireland. Many of the Irish names of myth that remain the most popular and appealing come from the Fenian legends. There's the princess Niamh, who ran away with Finn MacCool's son, Oisín; Gráinne, Finn's sweetheart, who eloped with Diarmaid; and Áine, who refused to sleep with any man but Finn. And on the male side, there are Diarmaid, Conán, Oisín and of course Finn MacCool himself, the quintessential hero with the quintessentially cool name.

Some other names of Irish legend are likewise well-used in modern times: Deirdre, for instance, Eithne, Maeve and Una for girls; Conor, Cormac and Ronan for boys. And there are names that survive only in legend that deserve to be revived: Caireann, Ceara, Daire and Marga are notable for their melodic qualities; and other names may inspire you because of their associations with mythical characters or events. Some other names of Irish legend survive as well: Deirdre, Eithne, Maeve, and Una for girls; Conor, Cormac, and Ronan for boys. There are also names that survive mainly in legend that deserve to be revived: Caireann, Ceara, Daire, and Glas are notable for their melodic qualities; Faife, Loch, and Torna sound distinctive and strong.

Another approach is to look for names that inspire because of their associations with specific characters and events. Etan is a daughter of the mythical god of healing, so might be perfect for a doctor's child. Aicher – or Ehir – was a legendary musician. But as inspirational as their original bearers may be, many of the names that follow should perhaps stay confined to legend. It's difficult to imagine a modern child going through life with the name Mongfind, for example, or Abhartach or Cuchulainn.

Here, for inspiration or maybe just for edification, is a who's who of Irish myth and legend:

Female

ACHALL
Daughter of the legendary warrior Cairbre Nia Fer; she died of sorrow when her brother was killed.

AÍ
Aí the Arrogant, daughter of Finn, who refused to marry any man who wasn't Irish. In keeping with her egotistical identity, her name is pronounced I.

AOIBHEALL
A pagan name of one of the ancient Irish goddesses. In various stories, she is the fairy who appears to Brian Boru on the eve of battle, the daughter of a warrior and the daughter of a king of Munster.

AILBHE
One legendary Ailbhe was a daughter of the fairy king Midir; another was a daughter of Cormac mac Art and one of the four best lovers in Ireland.

ÁINE

The name of many legendary heroines: a fairy queen; lover of the sea god who took her to the Land of Promise; daughter of the king of Scotland who would sleep with no man but Finn, whom she married and with whom she bore two sons.

AINNIR

A character in the Finn tales.

ALMHA

A member of the mythical tribe of divinities called the 'people of the goddess Dana', the legendary ancestors of the Irish race.

AOIFE

A warrior queen in love with Cúchulainn who bore him a son named Connla; the jealous stepmother in the Children of Lir tales. (The name began to rise in popularity after Siamese twins named Aoife and Niamh were successfully separated in 1997.)

BÁINE

Daughter of the legendary ancestor of Ireland's kings.

BANBHA

The name of an early Irish goddess who vied with sisters Fodla and Éire to have settlers name the country after them: obviously, Éire was the winner.

BEARACH

A character of legendary generosity, and the third wife of Finn.

BÉIBHINN

One legendary Béibhinn was the daughter of the king of the Otherworld; another was the mother of the hero slain by Cúchulainn.

BINNE

Name of several fairy-women of Irish legend.

BLÁTHNAIT

The wife of the Munster king Cú Rói and lover of Cúchulainn, whose life ended in tragedy; the word means 'little flower'.

BÓINN

Wife and mother of gods; goddess of the Boyne.

BRIGHID

A revered pagan goddess associated with poetry and fertility.

BUANANN

A goddess; also a mother who tutored warriors in arms.

CAINNLEACH

Foster mother of an Ulster hero, she died of sorrow when her son was slain.

CAIREANN

Daughter of the king of the Britons, mother of Niall of the Nine Hostages and legendary ancestress of the high kings of Ireland.

CATHACH

A legendary female warrior.

CEARA

A wife of a Nemed, a legendary invader of Ireland, who gave her name, Mac Cera to County Mayo.

CIARNAIT

Mistress of the legendary king Cormac mac Art.

CLÍODHNA

The name of three mythical heroines: a Tuatha Dé Danann, who gave her name to one of the three great waves of Ireland; one of the three beautiful daughters of Libra, poet to the sea god; and a fairy patroness to the MacCarthy clan.

CLOTHRA

Sister of legendary Queen Maeve.

COCHRANN

Mother of Diarmaid úa Duibne, the greatest lover in Irish legend, who eloped with Gráinne, Finn MacCool's beloved.

CRÉD

The name of several legendary queens and princesses, most notably the daughter of Cairbre, king of Ciarraige, who fell in love with the warrior Cáel and died of sorrow when he was slain in battle.

CRÓCHNAIT

Mother of the Fenian warriors Diarmaid and Oscar.

DÁIRINE

The daughter of a legendary king of Tara.

DANA/Danu

Pagan river goddess who bestowed her name on the Tuatha Dé Danaan, the legendary earliest inhabitants of Ireland.

DEIRDRE

Beautiful heroine of a tragic legend, who was betrothed to the king of Ulster but eloped with the young warrior Naoise, who was then killed by the king, after which the grieving Deirdre threw herself out of a chariot and died.

DELLA

Came to Ireland in a legendary invasion led by Queen Cessair.

DOIREANN

Daughter of the fairy king Midir.

DRAIGEN

Wife of the legendary ancestor of the kings of Munster.

DÚNLAITH

Daughter of the Connacht warrior Regamon; a popular name in the Middle Ages.

ÉABHA

A wife of Nemed, legendary invader of Ireland; also, a Fenian heroine who was drowned at sea.

EACHNA

Daughter of a king, she was reputed to be one of most beautiful and intelligent women in the world.

ÉIBHLEANN

A mythical spirit who gave her name to a mountain range.

ÉACHTACH

A daughter of the great lovers Gráinne and Diarmaid.

ÉILE

Sister of Queen Maeve.

ÉIRE

The victorious one of three sisters who competed to have Ireland named after her.

EITHNE

One of the most popular names of Celtic legend, in particular of the beautiful and clever Eithne, or Ethniu, who was imprisoned in a crystal tower and bore Lian's child Lugh, god of the sun and of arts and crafts.

EMER

Wife of the hero Cúchulainn, who stoically endured his acts of unfaithfulness. Appreciated for her six gifts – of beauty, voice, sweet speech, needlework, wisdom and chastity.

EÓRANN

A legendary queen, wife of Suibne.

ÉRNE

A princess after whom Lough Erne is named.

ÉTAÍN

One of several by this name was considered 'the most beautiful woman in all Ireland', but who, unfortunately, was turned by Midir's wife Fuamnach into a pool of water, a worm and a fly.

ETAN

The name of Cúchulainn's mistress as well as of the daughter of the mythical god of healing.

EVEGREN

Daughter of the tragic Deirdre and Naoise.

FAIFE

Daughter of Ailill and Queen Maeve.

FAÍLENN

A princess and the mother of Eithne, wife of the king of Cashel.

FAINCHE

One name of the Irish goddess of war; also a mythical saint who, when threatened with marriage, jumped into Lough Erne and swam underwater to the sea.

FANN

Wife of the sea god Manannán Mac Lir.

FÉTHNAT

Musician to the Tuatha Dé Danann.

FIAL

Wife of the founder of the O'Driscoll and O'Coffey families; also the name of Emer's sister and of a goddess.

FIDELMA

The name of several legendary queens, princesses and great beauties.

FINNABAIR

A daughter of Queen Maeve and Ailill.

FINNCHÁEM

The wife of Cian, the mother of the hero Conall Cearnach or the daughter of one fairy king and the wife of another.

FINNCHNES

In the Finn stories, the daughter of a king and also a robe maker for the Fianna.

FIONNUALA/Finnguala

The daughter of the sea god Lir, who was turned into a swan by her jealous stepmother Aoife and cursed to wander the lakes and rivers of Ireland.

FLIDAIS

Daughter of Ailill Finn, the legendary Connacht king, she fell in love with an exiled warrior.

FODLA

Wife of the god Mac Cecht whose name is another name for Ireland.

FUAMNACH

Wife of Midir, who in an act of jealousy turned her rival into a scarlet fly.

GRÁINNE

Finn MacCool's betrothed, who eloped with Diarmaid, and together they hid in forests and caves for sixteen years in what's considered one of the greatest love stories of Irish legend.

GRIAN

A daughter of Finn MacCool, possibly the Irish sun goddess.

ISEULT

Irish princess who was the lover of Tristan in the tragic Arthurian legend.

IUCHRA

She turned Aoife, her rival, into a heron.

LÍADAN

Mother of St Ciaran who, according to legend, conceived him when a star fell in her mouth; the poet beloved by Cuirithir.

LÍBAN

A mythical figure who lived beneath the sea for three hundred years.

LÓCH

Daughter of a legendary warrior and mother of the famous poet Nuadu Finn Éces.

LONNÓG

Noted for her kindness to Mad Sweeney, the mythical wild bird-man.

LÚGACH

A daughter of Finn MacCool.

MACHA

A war goddess of the Tuatha Dé Danann; another legendary Macha is called 'Macha of the red hair'.

MÁEN

Daughter of Conn of the Hundred Battles; another Máen was a king's daughter and mother of a legendary judge.

MARGA

Marga of the fairy mound was the mother of the beautiful but tragic Étain.

MÉADHBH/Maeve

The legendary Queen of Connacht who led an invasion of Ulster, which led to the death of Cúchulainn. The name means 'she who intoxicates'.

MELL

In Irish mythology, the mother of seven saints.

MUIREACHT

The wife of the king of Tara.

MUIREANN

Occurs frequently in Irish mythology: as Oisín's wife, the foster mother of the hero Cáel and the wife of a king of Connacht.

MUIRÍN

Lived for three hundred years in Lough Neagh.

MUIRNE

The mother of the great warrior Finn MacCool.

NEAMHAIN

An ancient war goddess.

NEASA/Nessa

The wily and ambitious mother of Conchobhar, responsible for bringing him to the throne.

NIAMH

Princess of the Land of Promise who left with Finn Mac-Cool's son Oisín for the Otherworld, where they lived happily for three hundred years.

ÓRLAITH/Orla

A name borne by both the sister and niece of Brian Boru.

SADB/Sive

Beautiful daughter of Conn of the Hundred Battles and wife of the legendary Munster king Ailill. Another Sadb was the mythical mother of Oisín who was transformed into a deer by a sorcerer.

SAMHAOIR

A daughter of Finn MacCool.

SÁRAIT

A legendary ancestress of the people of Muskerry and of the kings of Scotland.

SCÁTHACH

A female warrior and the teacher of Cúchulainn; another Scáthach lulls Finn to sleep with magic music.

SCOTA

The name of two progenitors of the Irish race, the wife of Niul and the wife of Milesius.

SUANACH

Sister of Finn MacCool and mother of the warrior Fiachra.

TAILLTE

A mythical nurse; also the wife of Eochaidh, the last king of the aboriginals of Ireland.

TEÁMHAIR

A mythical character after whom the Hill of Tara is named.

UNA

Daughter of a legendary king of Lochlainn and the mother of Conn of the Hundred Battles.

Male

AICHEAR

A musician of the Fianna.

AILBHE

The name of twelve warriors of the Fianna. Another mythical Ailbhe went seeking the Land of Promise.

AILILL

A warrior who fought a battle with the legendary Fothad, who had stolen his wife.

ÁINLE

An early sun god. Also, one of the three brothers who were slain by the king of Ulster, after he eloped with Deirdre.

AODH

This name appears frequently in Irish mythology and royal legend. One Aodh was a son of Lir, turned by Aoife into a swan.

BRAN

The name of two Fenian warriors as well as of Finn Mac-Cool's dog.

BREAS

A popular name in myth and legend.

BRIÓN

A name often found in very early legends, the most famous of which was the son of Echu Mac Énna, ancestor of the O'Connors, O'Rourkes, O'Flahertys, O'Reillys and other noble families.

CADHAN

A legendary hero who, with his dog, killed a monster.

CÁEL

A fallen Fenian hero, slain at the battle of Ventry.

CAÍLTE

A Fenian warrior famous for being swift of foot.

CAIRBRE

There are two legendary Cairbres: one was the son of Cormac mac Art; another Cairbre was the son of Niall of the Nine Hostages, founder of a royal dynasty.

CASS

A legendary ancestor of the Dál Cais, from whom the families O'Brien, MacNamara and O'Grady sprang.

CATHAIR

A legendary king of Leinster who had thirty-three sons.

CETHERN

A name for the god of the Otherworld; also father of a famous mythical Druid.

CIAN

The name of several legendary heroes, including the son of the god of medicine, who became father to Lugh, the sun god, the father of Ulster warrior Cúchulainn.

CIONNAOLA

In early law legends, a hero who remembered every word he learned at law school and wrote it down to form the first written record of Irish law.

CLOTHACH

Grandson of Dagda, the Good God.

CONAIRE

Name of a heroic high king, Conaire Már.

CONALL

The name of many legendary kings and heroes, including Conall Kernach, the great Ulster hero, and Conall Corc, founder of the kingship of Cashel.

CONÁN

Conán mac Mórna was a member of Finn MacCool's warrior band.

CONN

The name of a legendary king, Conn of the Hundred Battles, who is supposed to have been an ancestor of many famous families, including the O'Neills, the O'Donnells, the O'Rourkes, the O'Dowds and the O'Connors.

CONCHOBAR

In an Irish epic, Conchobar (modernised as Conor) mac Nessa, was the king of Ulster.

CORMAC

Legendary king of Tara, Cormac mac Art, who was ancestor of the O'Neills.

CRIOFAN

The name of several legendary kings and warriors.

CÚCHULAINN

The greatest of all the Irish warriors, hero of the Irish epic, *The Cattle Raid of Cooley* or *Táin Bó Cuailgne*.

CUMHAL

The father of Finn MacCool, or MacCúmhail, Cumhal mac Art was a king and champion of the west of Ireland, whose death in battle the day after his marriage was foretold by a Druid.

DAGDA

An imperial pagan god and leader of the legendary early inhabitants of Ireland.

DÁIRE

An early fertility god.

DÁITHÍ

A nephew of Niall of the Nine Hostages and a king of Connacht.

DIARMAID

A hero of Irish legend who fell in love with Gráinne, the beloved of Finn MacCool. He had a mark on his face that made women fall madly, instantly in love with him.

DONN

The god of the dead.

ÉIBHEAR

The son of Milesius; the name is an Irish version of the Latin Hibernia.

ÉNNAE

A legendary king of Munster.

EOCHAID

An extremely popular name in legend. One Eochaid was a lover of the fairy Étain.

FAERGHUS/Fergus

Fergus mac Róich was one of the heroes of the epic *The*

Cattle Raid of Cooley, famed for his strength and stamina; Fergus mac Erca was legendary leader of the Gaels' migration from Ireland to Scotland in the fifth century.

FEDELMID

The name of several mythological heroes, including the ancestor of the O'Neills.

FIACHNA

The son of a mythical sea god and brother of Fionnuala.

FIONN/Finn

Finn MacCool or Fionn mac Cúmhail, the greatest legendary hero of them all: leader of the Fianna, a band of thousands of warriors, musicians, poets, priests and physicians; acquired the gift of wisdom by touching the Salmon of Knowledge and sucking his thumb when he burned it cooking the fish; was the father of the master poet Oisín; spurned lover of Gráinne.

FÍTHEL

A legendary judge; also, a brother of Finn.

FRÁECH

The son of a fairy-woman, said to be the handsomest man in all Ireland and Scotland.

GAEL

Hero for whom the Irish race is named.

GLAS

Glas mac Aonchearda, a Fenian and follower of Finn MacCool.

LABHRAIDH

Labhraidh of the Red Hand was a Fenian hero who travelled with Oscar.

LÓCH

A mythological ancestor of the kings of Munster.

LUGH

Son of the goddess Eithne, known as 'master of all the arts'.

MIACH

A skilled craftsman, son of the pagan god Diancecht.

MIDIR

Fairy son of the god Dagda and lover of the beautiful Étain,

MORANN

A legendary judge of ancient Ireland who supposedly never gave an unjust verdict; also ten Fenian warriors.

MOROLT

Brother of Iseult, Tristan's doomed lover.

NAOISE

Deirdre's tragic lover.

NUADU

God of the Otherworld; the fisher-god.

ÓENGUS

Óengus of the Birds was the god of love and poetry among the pagan Irish.

OISÍN/Ossian

The son of Finn MacCool, he was the poet of the Fianna. He was married to Éibhir, but still managed to have a three-hundred-year alliance with Niamh Chinn Óir.

OSCAR

Finn MacCool's grandson, one of the great warriors of the Fianna.

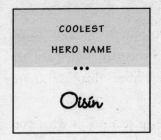

COOLEST
HERO NAME
...
Oisín

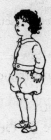

Africa

Irish Kings and Queens and Other Royalty

Until the twelfth century, when the Norman invaders finally got a stronghold in Ireland and the English king Henry II declared himself the country's overlord, Ireland was ruled by high kings as well as by a number of provincial kings and queens. The names of the most notable kings and queens – Brian Boru, Rory O'Connor, Gráinne O'Malley and the ancient queen Aoife, to name just a few – remain well used to this day. But there are many more ancient royal possibilities that are more obscure, and perhaps even cooler.

If raising a little Irish prince or princess is what you have in mind, look to this list for naming inspiration:

Female

ABHLACH

An Ulster princess and mother of a king.

AFRICA

Daughter of Fergus of Galway, who married Olaus the Swarthy, King of the Isle of Man.

AILBHE

Daughter of Cormac mac Art and mother of a warrior-king.

AILIONORA

Popularised by two queen consorts of England and introduced to Ireland by the Normans, the name was borne by several noblewomen.

AILLEANN

Two kings' mothers bore this name.

ÁLMATH

An early Ulster princess.

AOIBHINN

The name of several princesses, including a daughter of the royal prince of Tara who died in the tenth century.

AOIFE

Daughter of King Diarmaid of Leinster who married Strongbow, leader of the Norman invasion; also the name of many other princesses.

AURNIA

Wife of Turlogh More O'Brien, thirteenth-century king, this name is a variant of Orla.

BAILLGHEAL

A pious queen of Connacht.

BAIRRIONN

Wife of a twelfth-century Ulster king.

BEBHAILL

Queen of the high king Donnchad mac Aeda.

BEIBHINN/Bevin

Wife of Tadgh, tenth-century king of Connacht.

CAINNECH

Tenth-century princess.

CAOINTIARN

Two wives of high kings.

CEALLACH

Eighth-century princess. More common as a male name; gave rise to the last name O'Kelly.

CLODAGH

The name of a river popularised as a first name when the Marquis of Waterford gave it to his daughter.

COBHLAITH

A daughter of the powerful king Cano; also an eighth-century Leinster princess.

CRÉD

The name of several Irish queens and princesses, as well as of the mistress of Cano mac Gartnáin.

CRINOC

An eleventh-century Munster princess.

DAMHNAIT

Wife of a king of Munster and ancestress of the O'Moriartys, O'Cahills, O'Flynns and O'Carrolls.

DEARBHÁIL

The name of several medieval queens and princesses.

DERVOGILLA

The wife of Tiernan O'Rourke, king of Breifne; she eloped with Diarmaid McMurrough, king of Leinster, but later repented and became a nun.

DOIREANN/Dorren

The mother of Gilla Pátraic, an eleventh-century king.

DUIBHLEAMHNA

Daughter of a king and wife of a high king.

DÚNLAITH

Wife of the high king Niall Frassach as well as the name of daughters of two high kings.

EACHRA

A tenth-century princess noted for her beautiful complexion.

EIBHLÍN

A popular aristocratic name in Northern Ireland. It was brought to Ireland by the Normans in the forms Avelina and Emeline; is identical with the English Evelina and Evelyn; and – while it achieved popularity as Eibhlín – it has been retranslated as Eileen, Aileen and other variations.

EITHNE

The name of several early queens and princesses.

FAÍLENN

Wife of Cashel and mother of Eithne.

FINNEACHT

A princess of Meath and the mother of a saint.

FLANN

The name of two famous early queens; also a royal male name.

FORLAITH

A princess who became an abbess.

GORMLAITH

The name of several early and well-known queens, including the wife of high king Brian Boru, who was also a daughter of the king of Leinster and the mother of Sitric, king of Dublin.

GRÁINNE

Gráinne Mhaol Ni Mhaolmhaigh, or Grace O'Malley, was the

sixteenth-century queen of the Western Isles who is a poetic symbol of Ireland.

LASSAR
An early princess of Tara.

LÍOCH
The daughter of one high king and wife of another.

MAOL MHUADH
The name of several wives and daughters of kings and high kings.

MÓR
The name of several queens of Ireland.

MUIRGEL
The name of several queens of Leinster.

NÁRBHLA
The daughter of a prince and the wife of an abbot.

RANALT
Daughter of Awley O'Farrell, king of Conmacne, and wife of Hugh O'Connor, twelfth-century king of Connaught.

RÓNAIT
The daughter of a high king.

SADH
Daughter of Brian Boru, a queen of Connaught.

SÉADACH

An eleventh-century princess.

TAILLTE

Daughter of the king of Meath and wife of high king Turlough O'Connor.

TEMAIR

The wife of a seventh-century high king.

TUATHLA

An early queen of Leinster.

UALLACH

Chief poetess of Ireland in the tenth century.

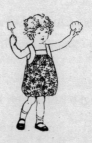

Male

AILILL

Ailill Molt, an early king.

AINMERE

Sixth-century king of Tara.

AODH/Hugh

The name of many kings and nobles, including three high kings.

ART

Art McMurrough, medieval king of Leinster.

AWLEY

Awley O'Farrell, king of Conmacne.

BAODÁN

The name of two powerful sixth-century kings.

BLATHMACC

A seventh-century king of Tara.

BRANDUBH

A medieval king of Leinster.

BREASAL

An early Leinster king.

BRIAN

Name of the most famous high king of Ireland, Brian Boru, who defeated the Norse.

CAILLÍN

An early prince who was ancestor to a dynasty of Cork kings.

CANO

A seventh-century king of Scotland and Ireland.

CATHAL

The name of a thirteenth-century king of Connacht, Cathal Crobhlhearg.

CEALLACHÁN

A tenth-century king of Munster.

CEARÚL

The name of a great warrior-king and of many noblemen of Leinster.

CEAT

King of Corcumroe; pronounced *Cat*.

CINÁED

An eighth-century high king, this name has been anglicised as Kenneth.

CINNÉIDE/Kennedy

King of Munster, father of Brian Boru.

CONALL

Conall Corc founded the kingship of Cashel.

CONCHOBAR

Conchobar (anglicisation: Conor) mac Nessa was king of Ulster.

CONGAL/Connell

A seventh-century Ulster king and an eighth-century high king.

CORMAC

Cormac MacCuilleanan, bishop and king of Munster. Also the name of several other kings, as well as the legendary ancestors of the O'Neills, O'Briens and MacNamaras.

CORMACÁN

One of the chief poets of medieval Ireland.

CRÍONÁN

An eleventh-century king and an ancestor of the O'Falveys.

CRUINN

An early king of Ulaid and the founder of a dynasty.

CUÁN

An early king; also an eleventh-century poet.

CUANA

An early warrior and the king of Fermoy.

DAITHI

A king of Tara.

DALLÁN

Two famous early poets.

DEÁMAN

An early Ulster king.

DIARMAID

Diarmaid MacMurrough was the twelfth-century Leinster king, who invited the Normans into Ireland.

DONNCHADH

High king and son of Brian Boru.

DONAL

The name of five high kings.

DÚNLANG

The name of two early kings, one who was an ancestor of the O'Donoghues and another who was an ancestor of the O'Tooles and O'Byrnes.

EOCHAID

An early Irish king, Eochaid Mugmedon, whose name means 'Lord of the Slaves'.

FAOLÁN

The name of three kings of Leinster between the seventh and ninth centuries.

FELIM

A medieval king of Connacht.

FERGUS

The name of several early kings.

FINGUINE

The name of two early Munster kings.

FLAITHRÍ

An early king; also an archbishop of Tuam and a distinguished ecclesiastic and writer.

FLANN

A distinguished name borne by a king, a high king, who was an ancestor of the O'Connors, and several famous early poets.

GLASSÁN

An early Ulster prince.

GORMAN

A king of Munster and an ancestor of the O'Keefes.

GUAIRE

A king of Connacht famed for his generosity.

LACHTNA

The name of several early kings and nobles, including the brother and the great-grandfather of Brian Boru.

LAOGHAIRE

A king of Tara.

LENNÁN

An early king.

LORCÁN

The name of several kings, including the grandfather of Brian Boru.

MAHON

Brian Boru's brother and a tenth-century king of Cashel.

MALACHY

The name of two famous high kings of Ireland.

MUIRÍOS

A favourite name among noble Connacht families.

MURTAGH

The name of three kings of Tara, as well as of the prince called Muircheartach of the Leather Cloak.

NIALL

King of Tara, Niall of the Nine Hostages, who founded the Ui Neill dynasty of Irish kings; also Niall Black-Knee, founder of the O'Neill family, who died fighting the Norse in the tenth century.

RUAIRÍ/Rory

Rory O'Conor, who ruled 1166–70, was the last high king of Ireland. Rory O'Donnell was the last king and first earl of Tyrconnell.

RUMANN

A great early poet.

SCANNLÁN

An early king.

SHANE

An Elizabethan era Irish prince, Shane the Proud, who was chief of the O'Neill family.

SITRIC

The name of several kings of Dublin in the Middle Ages, most notably Sitric Silkenbeard.

SUIBNE

An early high king.

TADGH

The name of several ancient kings and princes, including the son of Brian Boru, spelled Tadc.

TIBBOT

The son of Gráinne or Grace O'Malley, Tibbot of the Ship was so called because he was born at sea.

TURLOUGH

The name of two kings, Turlough I O'Brien and Turlough II O'Conor, who ruled in the tenth and eleventh centuries.

COOLEST
ROYAL NAME
• • •
Lennán

Tallula

Saints Preserve Us!

There are hundreds and hundreds of Irish saints, so many in fact that it seems as if every second person walking about the land in the fifth, sixth and seventh centuries must have been beatified. Not so surprising when you consider that Ireland was a centre of religious learning and fervour in those days, and sainthoods were also more generously conferred. And although many of their names live on only through the religious notoriety of their most famous bearers and are otherwise obsolete, there is a sizable group that are lovely and still appealing possibilities for twenty-first-century children. Here is a list of what we consider the coolest and most usable choices:

Female

NAME	OTHER/MODERN FORMS
ÁINE	*Anya, Enya*
AODHNAIT	*Enit, Ena, Eny*
ATTRACTA	
BLÁTH	*Flora*
BLINNE	*Moninne*
BREACNAIT	*Breccnat*
BRÍGH	*Brig, Bree*
BRIGID	*Bridget, Brid, Breda*
CAOILFHIONN	*Keelin, Kaylen*
CAOIMHE	*Keeva*
CEARA	*Cera, Keira*
CIAR	*Ciara, Kiara*
CLOTHACH	*Clora*
CONNA	
DÁIRE	*Darya, Dara*
DAMHNAIT	*Dymphna*
DANA	
DEARLÚ	
ÉADAOIN	*Aideen*
EITHNE	*Enya, Etna*
FAINCHE	*Fanchea*
FAOILEANN	*Failenn, Feelan*
FIDELMA	
FIONNAIT	*Fiona*
ÍDE	*Ida*

NAME	OTHER/MODERN FORMS
LALÓG	*Lallóc*
LÍADAN	*Líadaine, Lelia*
LONÁN	*Lonan*
LUÍSEACH	*Leesa*
MACHA	
MEADHBH	*Maeve*
MUADHNAIT	*Mona, Monat*
MUIRÍN	*Maureen*
NEAMH	*Neve, Ném*
ÓRNAIT	*Orna*
RÍONACH	*Rina, Riona*
SCIATH	*Skia*
SÉIGHÍN	*Séigíne, Shane*
TEAMHAIR	*Temair, Tara*
TUILELATH	*Tallulah*

Male

NAME	OTHER/MODERN FORMS
ABÁN	*Abbán*
AENGUS	*Angus*
AILBHE	*Alva*
AILLIL	
AODH	*Áed, Hugh*
AODHÁN	*Aidan*
AONGHUS	*Aengus, Angus*
BEAGÁN	*Beccán*

NAME	OTHER/MODERN FORMS
BRAN	
BRAON	*Breen*
BREACÁN	*Breccán*
BRENDAN	
BRÓGÁN	*Brogan*
CAOIMHÍN	*Kevin*
CASS	
CIANÁN	*Keenan*
CIARÁN	*Kieran*
CILLÍN	*Cillian, Killian*
COILEÁN	*Colin*
COLM	*Calam, Columb*
COLMÁN	*Colman*
CONALL	*Conal, Connell*
CONÁN	*Conan*
CONLAODH	*Conley*
CORCÁN	*Corccán*
CORCRÁN	*Corcoran*
CORMAC	
CRÍOFÁN	*Griffin*
CRÓNÁN	*Cronan*
CUÁN	
DÁIRE	*Dary*
DALLÁN	
DAMHÁN	*Daman, Davan, Davin*
DEAGLÁN	*Declan*
DIARMAID	*Dermot*

NAME	OTHER/MODERN FORMS
DONAL	*Donald*
DONNÁN	
DUFACH	*Duffy*
EARNÁN	*Ernan*
ELÁIR	*Alair*
EOGHAN	*Eoin, Owen*
EOLANN	*Olan*
EVIN	*Evan*
FAIRCHEALLACH	*Farrelly*
FAITHLEANN	*Fallon*
FAOLÁN	*Phelan*
FEARGHUS	*Fergus*
FINBARR	
FINNÉN	*Finian*
FINTAN/Fionntan	
FIONNÁN	*Finnán*
FLANN	
FLANNÁN	*Flannan*
GARBHÁN	*Garvin*
IODHAR	*Ibor, Ivor*
ÍOMHAR	*Ivor, Ifor*
LAOIRE	*Leary*
LORCÁN	*Lorcan*
LUCAN	
LUGHÁN	*Lugán*
MAC DARA	*MacDarra*
MAOL EOIN	*Malone*

NAME	OTHER/MODERN FORMS
MAOL MHUIRE	*Murray, Myles*
MAOLMHAODHÓG	*Malachy*
MEALLÁN	*Mellán, Mallon*
NAOMHÁN	*Nevan*
OISÍN	*Ossian*
ÓRÁN	*Oran*
PÁDRAIG	*Pádraic, Patrick*
RÍAN	*Rian, Ryan*
RODÁN	*Rodan*
RÓNÁN	*Ronan*
RÚADHÁN	*Rowan*
SEANÁN	*Senan, Shannon*
SIOLLÁN	*Sillán*
TADHG	*Tadc, Teague*
TIARNACH	*Tierney*
TIARNÁN	*Tiernan*
TRESSAN	*Tresian*

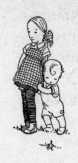

Holier By the Dozen

To multiply further the number of Irish saints, there are several names that count more than one saint to their credit. A lot more than one if ancient Irish records can be believed, for there are the following numbers of saints with these names:

COLMÁN	234	AODHAN/Aidan	21
FIONNTAN/Fintan	74	AODH/Hugh	20
MOCHUA	59	BRÉNAINNN/Brendan	17
MOLAISSE	46	BRIGIT	15
MO LUA	38	FAOLÁN	14
MOCHUMA	33	BRECCÁN/Breacán	13
COLUM	32	BRÍGH	13
CIARÁN	26		

Lugh

The Celticiser

In their search for a cool-sounding Irish name, some parents have begun to reverse the trend of anglicising traditional Gaelic names by going back to the originals or creating their own Irish-ised versions of Anglo names. Thus, if you wanted to honour your Grandpa Arnold, and couldn't find a direct Irish co-ordinate, you might fudge it by using something like Ardgal or Ardál instead. Here are some examples, but again, do feel free to improvise.

Girls

Angela	**AINGEAL**
Charlotte	**SÉARLAIT**
Clare	**CLÁR**

Claudia	**CLODAGH**
Edna	**EITHNE**
Eileen	**EIBHLÍN**
Evelyn	**AOIBHEANN**
Frances	**FAINCHE**
Grace	**GRÁINNE**
Gloria	**GIOLLA**
Helena	**LÉANA**
Isabel	**ISIBÉAL**
Louise	**LABHAOISE**
Mabel	**MÁIBLE**
Molly	**MAILLE/Mailsi**
Margery	**MAIREAD**
Patricia	**PÁDRAIGÍN**
Pauline	**PÓILÍN**
Polly	**PAILI**
Rachel	**RÁICHÉAL**
Sarah	**SARAID**
Sheila	**SÍLE**

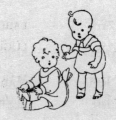

Boys

Alan	**AILÍN**
Albert	**AÍLBE** or **AILBHE**
Arnold	**ARDÁL**
Austin	**OISTIN**
Basil	**BREASAL**
Bernard	**BEARACH**
Calvin	**CEALLACHÁN/Calbhach/Calvagh**
Cary	**CARRAIG**
Conrad	**CONRÍ**
Dudley	**DUBHDARA**
Earl	**AEL**
Eugene	**EOGHAN/Eunan**
Emmett	**EIMÉID**
Gerald	**GEAROÍD**
Harold	**ARALT**
Jerome	**IAROM**
Kevin	**CAOIMHÍN**
Larry	**LABHRÁS**
Lew	**LUGH**
Mark	**MARCÁN**
Martin	**MÁIRTIN/Martán**

Peter	**PEADAR**
Raymond	**RÉAMONN**
Ronald	**RÓNAL**
Stephen	**STIOFÁN**
Steven	**STÉBHÍN**
Theodore	**THADÓIR**
Vincent	**UINSEANN**
Walter	**UALTAR**

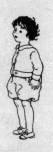

COOLEST

CELTICISED NAME

• • •

Mailsi

O'Duffy

Family Names

If you want a cool name from your family tree – but can't find any from recent generations for easy plucking – consider these choices traditionally used in various clans.

The good news is you can look back through names associated with all the various branches of your family to find some original and unexpected ideas. Don't forget too that families often dropped the prefixes Mac, Mc and O' over time, so if your family name is Kelly, you might consider O'Kelly family favourites Gráinne and Malachy, as your own.

The bad news is that there are many more names for boys here than for girls. Male names were more often passed down through a family, and also were more likely to be recorded, whereas female ones are often lost to time.

And many of these family names are, shall we say, a tad eccentric. Your heart may soar to spot your last name O'Madden on this list, only to feel it sink when you discover your family names are Anamcha, Breasal and Coganus. Such oddities may make better middle names than firsts. Some traditional names may be better left in the family graveyard. Awley Magawley? We don't think so.

We include both the Irish Gaelic and Anglicised forms of a name when both were used; when only one version is recorded, that's the one we include.

Girls

LAST NAME	FIRST NAME
Lowther	JANA
MacDermott	DERBHAÍL/Dervil
	FIONNUALA/Finola
	LASAIRIONA/Lasrina
MacDonagh	LASAIRIONA/Lasrina
MacMahon	BENVY
MacNamara	SLÁINE/Slany
MacNamee	GRÁINNE/Grania
McCourt	AISLING
O'Beirne	LASAIRIONA/Lasrina
O'Brien	CAOIMHINN
	FIONNUALA/Finola
	SLÁINE/Slany

O'Connor	**BENVY**
	ÉTAOIN
	FIONNUALA/Finola
O'Duffy	**GRÁINNE/Grania**
O'Flannagan	**ÉTAOIN**
O'Gormley	**GRÁINNE/Grania**
O'Hanley	**LASAIRIONA/Lasrina**
O'Hara	**ÉTAOIN**
O'Kane	**AISLING**
	RÓS/Rose
O'Kelly	**GRÁINNE/Grania**
O'Murray	**ROIS**
O'Neill	**BENVY**
Toler–Aylward	**ZINNA**
Wallis	**EDITHA**

Boys

LAST NAME	**FIRST NAME**
Barrett	**TOIMILIN**
Barry	**DOWLE**
Bradley	**AIBHNE/Eveny**
	MUIRCHEARTACH/Murtagh
Brady	**MAZIERE**
Brody	**AIBHNE/Eveny**
Burke	**FIACHA/Festus**
	UILLEAG
	UILLIAM/William

LAST NAME	FIRST NAME
Campbell	COILÍN/Colin
Clibborn	ABRAM
Dalton	PHILPOG
Fitzgerald	GEAROÍD/Garret
Foley	ENOG
Glenny	ÍOSAC/Isaac
Joyce	GILL
Kavanagh	ART
	DUNLANG/Dowling
	CRIOFAN/Griffin
	MURCHADH/Morgan
MacAlister	OENGUS/Angus
MacArdle	MALACHY
	RÉAMONN/Redmond
MacBrannon	CONN
	MAINE
MacBreen	MAINE
MacBrennan	AVERKAGH
MacCabe	AIRDGAL
MacCann	LOCHLAINN
	MALACHY
	COMHAI/Quinton
	RÉAMONN/Redmond
	RUAIDRÍ/Rory
MacCarten	ECHMHILIDH/Augholy/Eugenius

LAST NAME	FIRST NAME
MacCarthy	CEALLACHAN/Callahan
	DIARMAID/Dermot
	FININ/Florence
	JUSTIN
MacCawell	COMHAI/Quinton
MacClancy	BOETIUS
MacCloskey	MÁNUS
	COMHAI/Quinton
MacCormack	OENGUS/Aeneus
MacCoughlin	ROSS
MacDermott	GIOLLA CHRIOST/Christian
	MAOLRUANAI/Myles
MacDonagh	BRIAN
MacDonnell	OENGUS/Aeneus
	ALASTAR
	COLLA/Cole
	FEARDHACH/Frederick
	RANDAL
	RUAIRÍ/Rory
	SORLEY
MacDowell	ALASTAR
MacEgan	BEOLAGH
	LÚCÁS/Luke
	GIOLIA na NAOMH/Nehemias
MacElligot	UILLEAG/Ulysses
MacFaden	MANUS
MacGillespie	TÁRLACH/Charles

LAST NAME	FIRST NAME
MacGovern	BRIAN
	TIARNÁN
MacKenna	LOCHLAINN
MacKiernan	ART
	DUARCAN/Durkan
	TIARNÁN
Macken	RÉAMONN/Redmond
MacLoughlin	MUIRCHEARTACH/Murtagh
	OSCAR
MacMahon	AIRDGAL
	BRIAN
	CU ULLA/Cullo
	GLAISNE
	IRIAL
	COMHAI/Quinton
	ROSS
MacMasterson	DUARCAN/Durkan
MacMurrough	ART
MacNamara	CUMHEA/Cuvea
	MACCON
	SÍODA/Sheedy
MacNarnee	FARRELL
	LOCHLAINN
	SOLAM/Solomon
MacNicholl	MANUS
MacSweeney	TARLACH/Charles
	DUBHGHALL/Dougal
	EIREAMHÓN/Irwin
	EOGHAN

LAST NAME	FIRST NAME
Magawley	AWLEY
Magennis	ECHMHILIDH/Augholy/Eugenius
	ÉIBHEAR
	GLAISNE
Maguire	CU CHONNACHT/Constantine
	DONN
	OSCAR
	PILIB
	ROSS
Malone	LOCHLAINN
McGinley	RUAIRÍ/Rory
McRory	AIRDIN
Mulloy	RUAIRÍ/Rory
Nugent	BALTHASAR
O'Boyle	DUBHGHALL/Dougal
	FARRELL
O'Breslin	TARLACH/Charles
O'Brien	AINMIRE/Anvirre
	ANLUAN/Anlon
	BRAN
	CONCHOBAR/Connor
	DIARMAID/Dermot
	DONNCHADH/Donagh
	KENNEDY
	LAOISEACH/Lucius
	MUCHADH/Murrough
	TARLACH/Terence

LAST NAME	FIRST NAME
O'Brody	DAIRE
O'Byrne	FIACHA
	GARRETT-MICHAEL
	UGHAIRE
O'Carroll	MAOLRUANAI/Mulroney
O'Clerkin	FARRELL
O'Clery	CONAIRE
	LUGAID/Lewis
	TUATHAL/Tully
O'Connell	MUIRGHEAS/Maurice
	MURCHADH/Morgan
O'Connelly	AIRDGAL
O'Connor	ART
	BRIAN
	CALBHACH/Charles
	CONCHOBAR/Connor
	DIARMAID/Dermot
	EOGHAN/Owen
	FAILGHE
	MACBEATHA/MacBeth
	OSCAR
	RUAIDRI/Roderick
	TOMALTACH/Thomas
O'Daly	BAOLACH/Bowes
O'Dempsey	FINN
O'Dempster	FAILGHE
O'Doherty	CONALL
	RUAIRÍ/Rory
	TOIMILIN

LAST NAME	FIRST NAME
O'Donnell	AINEISLIS
	AODH/Hugh
	CATHBHARR/Caffar
	CONALL
	CONN
	EOGHAN
	MANUS
	NECHTAN
	NIALL/Neill
	RUAIRÍ/Rory
O'Donoghue	AMHLAOIBH/Auliffe
	SEAFRA/Geoffrey
O'Donovan	AINEISLIS
	MURCHADH/Morgan
O'Dowd	TOMÁS
O'Driscoll	FINN
	FOTHAD
	MACCON
O'Dunne	FAILGHE
O'Fallon	COFACH/Coganus
O'Falvey	DONNCUAN
O'Farrell	CEADACH/Kedagh
	CONMHAC/Canoc
	FACHTNA/Festus
	IRIAL
	ROSS
O'Flaherty	MAONACH
O'Flanagan	MALACHY

LAST NAME	FIRST NAME
O'Flynn	CU ULLA/Cullo
	COMHAI/Quinton
O'Gallagher	CONALL
	TARLACH/Charles
	TUATHAL/Tully
O'Gormley	SORLEY
O'Grady	STANDISH
O'Halloran	EIREAMHON/Erevan
O'Hanlon	RÉAMONN/Redmond
O'Hanly	BERACH/Barry
O'Hara	AILILL/Irril/Oliver
	CIAN/Kean
	DUARCAN/Durkan
O'Herlihy	CEALLACHAN/Callahan
O'Higgins	TUATHAL/Tully
O'Hogan	CRONEY
O'Kane	AIBHNE/Eveny
	ECHLIN
	JARMY
	MANUS
	COMHAI/Quinton
O'Keeffe	CORC
	FINGUINE
	GORMAN
O'Kelly	BREASAL
	BRINE
	FERADACH

LAST NAME	FIRST NAME
O'Kelly (cont)	FIACHA/Festus
	LOCHLAINN/Laurence
	MALACHY
	MAINE/Many
	NIALL/Neill
	UILLIAM/William
O'Kennedy	DONN
O'Lafferty	EIBHEAR
O'Lohan	AMHRA
O'Loughlin	IRIAL
O'Madden	ANAMCHA/Ambrose
	BREASAL
	COFACH/Coganus
O'Mahoney	CIAN/Cain
	FININ
	MAOL MHUIRE/Molloy
O'Mara	ELAN
O'Meehan	MOLAISSE/Lazarus
O'Molloy	UAITHNE/Greene
	CEADACH/Kedagh
O'More	CONMHAC/Canoc
	FACHTNA/Festus
	RUAIRÍ/Roger
O'Moriarty	CORC
	SEANCHEN/Jonathan
O'Morgan	MALACHY
O'Mullin	AIBHNE/Eveny

LAST NAME	FIRST NAME
O'Mulloy	ART
O'Neill	CONN
	CU ULLA/Cullo
	ENRI
O'Nolan	UGHAIRE
O'Quinn	NIALL/Neill
O'Reilly	FAILGHE
	GLAISNE
	MYLES
O'Rourke	ART
	CONN
	FEARGHAL/Farrell
	TIARNAN
O'Shaughnessy	RUAIRÍ/Roger
O'Sullivan	BUADACH/Boethius
	FININ
O'Toole	BARNABY
	DONNCUAN
	GILKEVIN
	LORCAN
Parsons	SAVAGE
Reynolds	IOR
Trant	ION
Tyrrell	PHILPOG
Wall	UILLEAG/Elias
Ward	MANUS

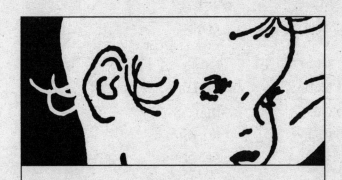

IV. NEW COOL

...

Creative Names

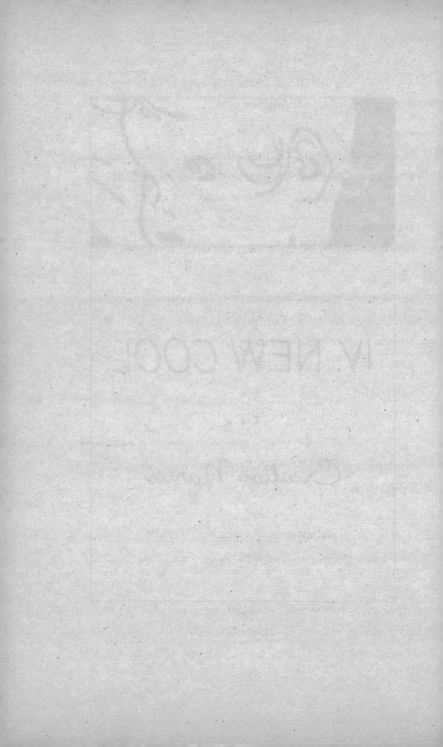

Donegal

Cool Irish Place Names

From Tipperary to Tralee, Irish names are melodic and evocative. Some of the selections on this list may strike you as thoroughly feminine, others strongly masculine, but most, we think, could work well for children of either sex.

Names of Irish towns, countries, rivers and hills, both real and imaginary, that have been or could be used for both boys' and girls' first names include:

ADARE	ARDNAREA
ARAN	ARLESS
ARBOE	ARMAGH
ARDAGH	ATHY
ARDARA	BALLA
ARDEE	BALLINA

BARROW	DURROW
BOHO	EALGA
BOYLE	EMLY
BOYNE	ENNIS
BRAY	FINN
CARLOW	FINNEA
CARRA	GALWAY
CARRICK	GLIN
CARY	GYLEEN
CASHEL	IERNE
CASHEN	INISHEER
CAVAN	JUVERNA
CLARE	KAVANAGH
CLAREEN	KERRY
CLIFDEN	KILCLARE
CLODAGH	KILDARE
CLOONE	KILKENNY
CONNEMARA	KILLALA
CONNOR	KILLEIGH
CORBALLY	KILLIAN
CULLEN	KINSALE
CURRAGH	LEENANE
DERRY	LEIGHLIN
DONEGAL	LIFFEY
DOON	LOUGHLIN
DUBLIN	LUCAN
DUFFERIN	MAGHERA
DULANE	MAHEE

MALLOW	SHANNON
MANULLA	SLANE
MAYO	SLIGO
MEADE	SUIR
MONAGHAN	SUTTON
NAVAN	TARA
OMAGH	TEMPO
OOLA	TIAQUIN
PALLAS	TORY
QUIN	TRALEE
RAHAN	TULLA
RAMONE	TYRELLA
ROSS	TYRONE
SAMHAOIR	VALENTIA
SCOTA	VARTRY
SHANDON	WICKLOW

COOLEST
PLACE NAME
• • •
Donegal

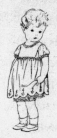

Lennon

Cool Last Names

Last names used as first names are generally hip, but Irish family names – and the Irish were among the first cultures to use more than one name – have a special blend of spirit and tradition that has made them particularly adaptable as first names, used all over the English-speaking world. We're all familiar with Ryan and Kelly, Casey and Clancy, Barry and Blake, but there are countless others waiting to be discovered and switched into first position. Here are a few ideas, with an element of their coolness, but by all means feel free to comb through the branches of your own family tree.

BAILEY

Spreading like wildfire through the USA and catching spark in London as a first name for both boys and girls.

BAKER

Occupational last-name names are a hot new category.

BANNAN

A name connected to one of the most famous haunted castles in Ireland.

BEHAN

A literary name strongly associated with acclaimed playwright Brendan Behan.

BOYLAN

A fourteenth-century poet praised the Boylans for their horsemanship and blue eyes.

BRENNAN

A more modern-sounding spin on the traditional favourite Brendan.

CALLAGHAN/Callahan

Might be a twin name with Kelly, as they both derive from Ceallach.

CASSIDY

Has taken on a cowboy image, thanks to American 1950s western icon, Hopalong Cassidy.

CLOONEY/Cluny

Meaning 'grassy meadow' or 'sexy international superstar'.

CONELLY/Conolly

A Donegal lawyer named William Conolly (1662–1729) was, in his day, reputed to be the richest man in Ireland.

CONNERY

Strongly associated with the super-suave James Bond, Scottish-born Sean Connery.

CONROY

A distinguished Irish last name connected for generations with hereditary poets and chroniclers to the kings of Connacht.

CONWAY

Notable Conways have included eminent religious, military and scientific figures.

COONEY

It comes from the Irish 'cuanna', which means 'handsome or elegant'.

CORRIGAN

The family motto is 'Wisdom and impetuosity' – a very cool combination.

CREA

Can be used on its own, or as its patronymic, McCrea.

CROSBY

Gained international fame via nonchalant crooner Bing Crosby.

CULLEN

Ireland's first Cardinal was Cardinal Paul Cullen of County Kildare.

CURRAN

Unusual and savoury name, conjuring up images of curry and currants.

DEEGAN

A very old name meaning 'son of the black-haired one'.

DENNISON

A cooler namesake for Grandad Dennis.

DOLAN

Fresh choice to replace Dylan or Nolan.

DONNELLY

Has lots of rhythmic three-syllable energy.

DONOGHUE/Donahue

Brian Boru, the most famous of the high kings, had a son with this name.

DUFFY

Slightly rowdy feel, would be right at home in a noisy pub.

DUGAN

Open, friendly and cheerful.

EGAN

Its likeness to the word 'eager' gives Egan a ready-to-please, effervescent energy.

FINNEGAN

Tied to one of the great works of Irish literature, *Finnegan's Wake*.

FLAHERTY

A name borne by several early Irish kings.

FLANAGAN

Has a warm, cosy, flannelly feel.

FLYNN

Like Flann and Flanagan, suited to a redhead.

GALLAGHER

Good for a future traveller, as it means 'lover of foreigners'.

GILLIGAN

Cool despite connection to dorky American TV character.

HOGAN

Cool first-name possibility, à la Scottish Logan.

KAVANAGH/Cavanaugh

A substantial surname that moves beyond Casey and Cassidy.

KEENAN

In the Middle Ages, the Keenans were distinguished ecclesiastics and historians.

KENNELLY

A contemporary-feeling namesake for an ancestral Kenneth.

LANIGAN

Found mostly in Kilkenny, Tipperary and Limerick, would make a lively choice.

LENNON

Has already started to be used as a baby name in tribute to Beatle John.

LONERGAN

The Lonergans have both an ecclesiastical and musical heritage.

LOWRY

Admirable family motto: 'Virtue evergreen'.

MACCORMAC

More unusual than its offshoot, Cormac.

MACCOY

A boy with this name would indeed be the real MacCoy.

SOME MORE APPEALING
MAC NAMES

• • •

MACAULEY	MACDONAGH	MACHUGH
MACBIRNEY	MACDONALD	MACKEEVER
MACCABE	MACDONNELL	MACNEELEY
MACCLURE	MACGARRY	MACNIELL
MACCOLUM	MACGLYNN	MACQUADE

MACDERMOT
Dating back to twelfth-century King Dermot of Moylurg, they were the only Irish family to have a princely title.

MACSWEENEY
See Sweeney.

MAGEE
Though it means 'Son of Hugh', Magee would have a broad and bouncy appeal for any Dad's son.

MAGUIRE
This common last name has a lot of verve as a first.

MALONE
Classic last name with a lot of character.

MOLLOY
The title of a Samuel Beckett novel.

MOONEY
A name with two possible meanings: 'dumb' or 'wealthy'. We'll opt for wealthy.

MOORE
Would make an elegant middle name.

MORRISSEY
Indie singer/songwriter (Steven Patrick) Morrissey made this a viable first name option.

MURPHY

It actually started life as a first name meaning 'warrior of the sea'.

NOLAN

This one's already entered the first-name column.

NUGENT

The term to 'nugentise' dates back to poet Robert Nugent, who sustained himself by marrying wealthy widows to the point where he was able to lend money to King George III.

O'BRIEN

Based on the name of Brian Boru, the legendary tenth-century High King of Ireland and perfect for the grandson of a Brian.

O'CONNOR

Last name of countless eminent writers, entertainers, politicians and diplomats.

O'GRADY

An American O'Grady was the great-grandfather of boxing immortal Muhammed Ali.

O'NEILL

Associated with the prominent American playwright Eugene O'Neill.

QUINN

Shades of 'The Mighty Quinn' – a movie, a band and a Bob Dylan song.

RAFFERTY

Already coolised by Jude Law and Sadie Frost as the name of their son.

REDMOND

Has a dash of danger, thanks to infamous highwayman Redmond O'Hanlon.

REAGAN/Regan

US President Ronald Reagan was one of many distinguished descendants of Brian Boru.

REILLY/Riley

A huge unisex hit in the USA.

RIORDAN/Reardan

Originated as a profession name for a royal poet.

ROONEY

Light-hearted name with meaningful meaning: 'descendant of the hero'.

SCULLY

You can pat yourself on the back with this name meaning 'descendant of a scholar'.

SHANAHAN

Has a lot more bounce and masculine dash than Shannon ever did.

SHERIDAN

Name of one of Ireland's wittiest playwrights, Richard Brinsley Sheridan.

SULLIVAN

Has a real twinkle in its eye.

SWEENEY

An upbeat name that appears in the works of Yeats, TS Eliot and Flann O'Brien – not to mention Sweeney Todd.

TIERNAN

The original Tiarnán was the name of early chieftains, kings and princes.

TIERNEY

Like cousin Tiernan, a cool choice for either girls or boys.

COOLEST
SURNAME NAME
•••
O'Brien

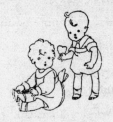

Breege

Cool Nicknames

For the first time since the 1960s, nicknames have become a hot category of baby names, mostly those that are older, funkier diminutives with a Victorian pedigree. It's a trend that started in England but is quickly gathering momentum elsewhere, with some of the names already having jumped on the Irish popularity polls. Among those you can consider putting directly on the birth certificate:

Girls

ABBIE/Abby	AGGIE
ADDIE	BEA

BEESY	KITTY
BERNIE	LETTY
BIDDY	LIL
BREE	LOTTIE
BREEGE	LULU
BRID	MAIDIE
BRIDIE	MAISIE
CAIT	MAMIE
CASSIE	MO
CLEO	NELLY
COCO	NONIE
DAISY	PAILI
DETTA	PEIG
DIXIE	PEIGÍ
DOTTIE	POLLY
EDIE	PRU
EILY	RENNY
ELLIE	ROSIE
EMMY	SADIE
EVIE	SAM
FLORRIE	SIBBY
GRACIE	SUKEY
IZZY	TESSIE
JAZ	TILLIE
JOSIE	TRIONA
KAT	
KATIE	
KIT	

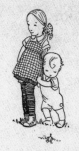

Boys

ALF	JOE
ALFIE	JOHNNY
ARCHIE	KIT
AUGIE	LACHIE
BARNEY	LOUIE
BAZ	MAC
BEC	MICK
BENNO	MOSS
BILLY	NED
BRAN	NEILIE
BRY	OLLIE
CHARLIE	OZZIE
CHRISTY	PADDY
CON	RAY
DEZ	SÉIMÍ
DEZI	SHAY
DONN	SULLY
EOCHO	THAD
FLURRY	THEO
FREDDY	TOM
GEORGIE	TULLY
GUS	WILL
JAMIE	

Carraig

Irish Word Names

One of the coolest trends in the USA, now extending to other languages as well, is word names: simply, words that, because they have a wonderful meaning and an appealing sound, make for fresh, evocative names. There's no reason this idea can't be translated into Irish as well. Here, some ideas for Irish words that might work as names. But this is just a beginning. Your imagination, and your dictionary, are the limit.

ABHAINN	river
BRONNTANAS	gift
CARRAIG	rock
CEART	justice

EALA	swan
ÉAN	bird
EARRACH	spring
EILIT	doe
FEILEACÁN	butterfly
FEOTHAN	breeze
FIA	deer
FÍRINNE	truth
FOMHAIR	autumn
GEALACH	moon
GEIMHREADH	winter
MUINÍN	trust
NEAMH	heaven
RÉALTA	star
SAIBREAS	wealth
SAMHRADH	summer
SEODRA	jewel
SÍOCHÁIN	peace
SPÉIR	sky
TAILBREAMH	dream
TONN	wave

Laoise

Names with Cool Meanings

Nature names, animal names and names with uplifting or exciting meanings are cool in any language. A selection of Irish names with interesting meanings:

Girls

ÁINE – radiance, splendour, brilliance

AISLING – dream, vision

AOIFE – beautiful, radiant

AOIBHEANN – radiant beauty

BLÁTHÍN – blossom

CAOIMHE – comely, beautiful

CASS – curly haired

CARMEL – garden

CATRIONA – pure
CROEB – branch, garland

DANA/Danu – abundance, wealth
DYMPHNA – a fawn

EIBHLÍN – wished-for child
EINÍN – little bird

FIAMAIN – swift-footed creature
FIONNUALA – white shoulders
FÍONA/Fina – vine
FÍRINNE – truth

GEILÉIS/Gelace – bright swan
GRIAN – sun

KEELY – graceful

LAOISE – radiant girl
LASAIR – flame

MAIRÉAD – pearl
MUÍRGHEAL – bright as the sea

NIAMH – radiance, brightness
NONÍN – daisy

ÓRLA – golden princess
OSNAIT – little deer

PÁDRAIGIN – noble

REALTÁN – star
RÓISÍN – little rose

SAOIRSE – freedom

SCOTH – bloom, blossom

SIBÉAL – wise woman

SÍLE – pure and musical

SÍOMHA – peace

SIVE – sweetness, goodness

SLÁINE/Slany – health

SORCHA – radiant

TEAGAN – beautiful

TUATHLA – princess of the people

Boys

AEDAL – highly courageous

ANBHILE – great tree

AODH – fire

AONGHUS – vigour

ART – bear

BRADEN – salmon

BROCK – badger

CADHAN/Kyne – wild goose

CANA/Cannagan – wolf cub

CLOONEY – grassy meadow

COLM/Colum – dove

CONÁN – great, high

CURRAN – hero, champion

DARRAGH – like an oak
DECLAN – full of goodness

EILTÍN/Eltin – young deer, lively person

FERGAL – valiant

LENNÁN – sweetheart, lover
LONÁN – blackbird
LONEGAN – bold, fierce

MARCÁN – steed
MUGHRÓN – lad of the seals

PEADAR – rock
PHELIM – constant

OISÍN/Ossian – little deer
OSCAR – deer lover

QUINLAN – of beautiful shape

RONAN – little seal

SEÁN – God's gracious gift
SORLEY – summer wanderer

TADGH – poet, philosopher

Addisyn

Newbies

Here, hot off the press from newspapers across the country, are what Irish parents are choosing to name their newborns now:

Girls

ABBI	ANNALIE
ADA	AOIBHNE
ADDISYN	AOIFE
AILBHE	ARABELLA
AISLING	AVA
AISLINN	BEATRICE
ALANNA	BERNADETTE
ALICE	BLÁTHNAID
AMELIA	CAMILLE
AMELIE	CAOIMHE

CARAGH	LUDMILLA
CIANNA	LULU
CIARA	MAEVE
CLARA	MIA
CLARE	MUIREANN
CLODAGH	NESSA
EÁBHA	NIAMH
EIMEAR	NICOLA
EITHNE	NORA
ELAINA	OLIVE
ELIZA	OLIVIA
EVA	ÓRLA
EVIE	ÓRLAITH
FAY	PHILOMENA
FIA	RÓISÍN
FIONA	RUBY
GRACE	SADBH
GRÁINNE	SAMARA
HARRIET	SAOIRSE
IONA	SASHA
ISABEL/Isabelle/Isobel	SIOBHAN
JULIET	SIÚN
LAOISE	SOPHIE
LARAGH	SORCHA
LEEANNA	TAMSIN
LIBBY	TARA
LILIAN	THALIA
LUCIA	ZARAH
LUCY	ZOE

Boys

AIDAN	FIONN
AILBHE	FLYNN
ALFIE	FREDDY
ARAN	GARETH
ARCHIE	GARVAN
BENEDICT	HARRY
CALEB	HARVEY
CALLUM	HUGH
CIAN	HUGO
CILLIAN	ISAAC
CLEMENT	JACK
CONN	JARLATH
CONOR	JUDAH
CORMAC	JUDE
CÚAN	KEALAN
DÁIRE	KILLIAN
DECLAN	LEO
DIARMUID	LOCHLAINN
DYLAN	LUKE
EAMON	MAX
ÉNÁN	MURROUGH
EOIN	NATHAN
FABIEN	NED
FIACHRA	NIALL
FINLAY	NOEL
FINN	ODHRÁN

OISÍN

ORAN

OSCAR

PADDY

PADRÁIG

RIAN

RONAN

RORY

RUADHÁN

SEAMUS

SEBASTIAN

SENAN

TADHG

THEO

TIARNÁN

TIERNAN

TOBY

TORLOUGH

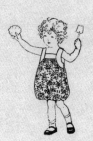

Pronunciation Guide for Irish Names

The guide below might look a little daunting (and this book is supposed to be fun!), but if you have selected that special name for your baby and want to make sure you are pronouncing it correctly then read on. Capitals denote the syllable in a name that should be stressed. Please note that there are different subtleties and inflections for many of the names – here we have attempted to show the Irish pronunciation for each.

The Irish Alphabet

VOWELS

There are two types of vowels in Irish:

Short Vowels		Long Vowels	
a	like English **a** tap	á	like English **awn** in awning
e	like English **e** in get	é	like English **e** in hey
i	like English **i** in pit	í	like English **ee** in knee
o	like English **o** long	ó	like English **o** in woe
u	like English **u** in tug	ú	like English **oo** in cool

VOWEL COMBINATIONS (Dipthongs)

This is the most awkward part of Irish pronunciation, when two vowels come together. The table below shows how these combinations are pronounced.

Long Dipthongs

Written	Pronounced	Sample	Pron.
ae	Eng. 'tray'	Ir. Gael (Irish person)	*gayle*
ao	Eng. 'tree'	Ir. maor (steward)	*mweer*
eo	Eng. 'Joe'	Ir. ceo (fog)	*keyo*
ia	Eng. 'see a'	Ir. nia (nephew)	*knee-a*
ua	Eng. 'truant'	Ir. tua (axe)	*Too-a*
ea	Eng. 'mass'	Ir. meas (respect)	*mass*
io	Eng. 'miss'	Ir. pionta (pint)	*pin-ta*
ui	Eng. 'quiz'	Ir. puinn (not much)	*pwin*

CONSONANTS

Traditonally, the Irish Alphabet consists of the following consonants:

b c d f g h l m n p r s t

Consonants are pronounced in relation to the vowels around them. In Irish 'i' and 'e' are called slender vowels and 'a', 'o' and 'u' broad vowels. 'C', followed by 'a', 'o' and 'u', is broad, whereas 'C' followed by 'e' or 'i' is slender, therefore the name Cathal is pronounced Cah-hal and Cillian is KIL-e-an.

There are fewer consonants in Irish than there are in English, and in a number of cases, as the examples below show, the Irish and English are quite similar.

Broad Consonant	Example	English Equivalent
b	**b**ád (boat)	**b**at
c	**c**óta (coat)	**c**oat
d	**d**oras (door)	**d**oor
f	**f**an (wait)	**f**an
g	**g**úna (dress)	**g**ood
l	**l**ampa (lamp)	**l**amp
m	**m**ála (bag)	**m**atch
n	gú**n**a (dress)	**n**ap
p	**p**ota (pot)	**p**ot
r	**r**ás (race)	**r**ash
s	**s**alach (dirty)	**S**ally
t	**t**olg (sofa)	**t**alk

Slender Consonant	Example	English Equivalent
b	**b**ille (bill)	**b**ill
c	**c**ill (church)	**k**ill
d	**d**il (drop)	**J**ill
f	**f**ill (return)	**Ph**il
g	**g**ile (brightness)	**g**irl
l	**l**ig (let)	**l**ick
m	**m**ill (ruin)	**m**ill
n	**n**igh (wash)	**n**ine
p	**p**ictiúr (picture)	**p**ick
r	**r**ith (run)	**r**inse
s	**s**íl (think)	**sh**in
t	**t**ine (fire)	**ch**in

ASPIRATION

Some consonants in Irish can undergo a transformation called *séimhiú*, which is sometimes translated as *aspiration*. This is represented by putting the letter 'h' after the consonant. This changes the pronunciation of the consonants, and naturally there is both a broad and a slender version for each. This can happen at the beginning, the middle or the end of a word.

Aspirated consonants

Broad Pronounced/example

bh	Eng. 'w'
ch	As in 'loch'
dh	Like 'ch' but based on a 'g' sound
fh	Silent
gh	Like 'ch' but based on a 'g' sound
mh	Eng. 'w'
ph	Eng. 'f'
sh	Eng. 'h'
th	Eng. 'h'

Slender Pronounced/example

bh	Eng. 'v'
ch	Like the broad consonant
dh	Eng. 'y'
fh	Silent
gh	Eng. 'y'
mh	Eng. 'v'
ph	Eng. 'f'
sh	Eng. 'h'
th	Eng. 'h'

Aalin *AH-lin*
Aamor *AH-moore*
Abán *Ah-BAWN*
Abbán *Ah-BAWN*
Abhainn *Ah-WAN*
Abhlach *av-lah*

Abram *AY-bram*
Achall *AH-hill*
Ada *AY-da*
Adare *Ah-dare*
Adaryn *Ah-darin*
Adeon *AH-dion*

Adigis *AH-digis*
Ado *AEdo*
Adolphus *Ah-DOL-fus*
Áed *Aid*
Aedal *Aid-al*
Ael *AH-eel*

Aela *Ay-la*
Aelwen *Ay-EL-wen*
Aeneus *Aynus*
Aerona *Ay-rona*
Aibhne *AV-nya*
Aichear *Acre*
Aideen *ay-DEEN*
Ailbhe *AISLE-va*
Ailill *AL-eel*
Ailín *AL-een*
Ailionóra *ALLY-oh-nora*
Ailleann *ALL-yan*
Aillila *AL-eel-a*
Ailsa *AISLE-sa*
Áine *AH-nya*
Aineislis *An-E-S-lis*
Aingeal *ANG-gil*
Ainle *AN-la*
Ainmere *An-mare*
Ainmire *An-mira*
Ainnir *AN-yir*
Ainnle *AN-la*
Airdgal *Ard-gal*
Aisling *Ashling*
Aislinn *Ashlen*
Alair *AY-lare*
Aled *A-lid*
Aleel *AL-eel*
Alef *A-lef*
Alienor *Ai-LIN-or*
Álmath *AL-math*
Almeda *AL-meda*
Almha *AL-wa*
Amaryllis *Am-ar-ILLIS*
Amatheon *Ah-MATH-eon*
Amelie *Am-a-lee*
Amhlaoibh *OW-lee*
Amhra *OW-ra*
Anamcha *AN-am-ha*
Anarawd *AN-ar-wid*
Anbhile *AN-vile*
Anchoret *AN-chore-et*
Aneira *An-EAR-ra*
Aneurin *An-YOUR-in*
Angharad *An-GA-ra*
Angwyn *ANG -gwin*

Anluan *AN-loo-an*
Anun *AH-noon*
Aodh *Ay*
Aodhán *AY-gan*
Aodhnait *EE-nitch*
Aoibhe *E-va*
Aoibheall *E-val*
Aoibheann *EE-van*
Aoibhinn *EE-veen*
Aoibhne *EVE-nya*
Aoife *EE-fa*
Aoirghe *EARr-ge*
Aonghus *AING-gus*
Aralt *AH-ralt*
Aravis *AH-ra-vis*
Arboe *AHR-bo*
Ardagh *AHR-da*
Ardal *AHR-dal*
Ardan *AHR-den*
Ardara *AHR-dara*
Ardee *AHR-dee*
Ardnarea *Ard-NAR-ea*
Ariadne *Ahr-ree-ad-nee*
Arless *Ar-less*
Armagh *Ar-MA*
Aroon *AH-roon*
Arwen *Ar-win*
Athol *Ah-tall*
Athy *A - THIGH*
Augholy *AWE-hully*
Aurnia *Our-NEE-a*
Auron *OUR-on*
Austell *OS-tell*
Averkagh *A-VER-ka*
Ayamonn *Eye-A-mon*
Azenor *AH-zen-ore*

Baillgheal *Bwill-YALL*
Báine *BAN-ah*
Baird *Bardge*
Bairrfhionn *BAR-in*
Bairrionn *BAR-in*
Ballina *Ball-IN-ah*
Banadel *BAN-a-dell*
Banbha *Ban-va*
Baodán *Bway-DAWN*
Baolach *BWAY-la*

Barrdhubh *BARR-goo*
Bartell *BAR-tel*
Beagán *Bug-AWN*
Bearach *BAR-ak*
Bebhaill *BAY-vill*
Beccán *Beck-AWN*
Beesy *Bee-see*
Behan *BEE-han*
Béibhinn *BAY-vin*
Benvy *Ben-vee*
Beolagh *Bee-OH-la*
Berach *BEAR-ah*
Beriana *Bear-EE-ana*
Berwin *Bear-win*
Binne *Bin-ya*
Bláth *BlAW*
Bláthín *BLAW-heen*
Blathmacc *BLA-mac*
Bláthnaid *BLAW-nidge*
Bláthnait *BLAW-natch*
Blinne *BLIN-ya*
Blodwen *BLOD-win*
Boetius *Bo-it-EE-us*
Bóinn *BO-in*
Boylan *BOY-lin*
Boyne *Boyin*
Brandubh/Branduff
   Bran-DUFF
Braon *Brain*
Brastius *BRAS-tee-us*
Breacán *Brack-AWN*
Breacnait *BRACK-nitch*
Breas *Bras*
Breasal *Bras-al*
Breccán *Brek-AWN*
Breccnat *Brek-nat*
Brecon *Brek-on*
Breda *BREE-da*
Breizh *Brez*
Brénainnn *BRAY-nan*
Brid *Breedge*
Bridge *Breedge*
Bridie *BRIDE-ee*
Brígh *Bree*
Brión *BREE-on*
Bronntanas *BRUN-tan-is*

Brynna *BREE-anna*
Buadach *BOO-da*
Buanann *BOOAN-an*
Buchanan *Bew-can-an*

Caden *Cadin*
Cadhan *KYE-in*
Cadoc *CAH-doc*
Cáel CAH-el
Caillín *Calleen*
Cailte *CAYIL-cha*
Cainnech *KAN-ya*
Cainnleach *KAN-lac*
Cairbre *CAR-bray*
Caireann *Car-in*
Cait *Catch*
Caitlin *CATCH-lean*
Calam *Cal-am*
Calbhach *CAL-wa*
Caleb *KAY-leb*
Callaghan *KAL-a-han*
Calvagh *CAHL-va*
Campbell *CAHM-bell*
Cana *CAH-na*
Cannock *CAN-ock*
Caoilfhionn *KALE-inn*
Caoilinn *KALE-een*
Caoimhe *Key-va*
Caoimhín *KEY-veen*
Caointiarn *KEEN-cheern*
Caradoc *CAR-a-dock*
Caragh *CAR-a*
Carantec *Car-AN-tec*
Carraig *Car-ig*
Cashel *Cash-il*
Caswallawn *KAS-wal-on*
Cathach *Caha*
Cathair *CAH-hir*
Cathal *Cah-hal*
Cathbharr *CAH-war*
Catriona *Cat-TREE-na*
Cavan *Cah-van*
Ceadach *KYA-da*
Ceallach *Kyalla*
Ceallachan *KYALLA-han*

Ceara *KEER-a*
Ceart *Keyart*
Cearúl *KAR-ool*
Céat *Kate*
Céibhionn *KAY-vin*
Cera *Kera*
Ceridwen *KER-id-win*
Cerys *Sir-EES*
Cethern *KETH-ern*
Cian *Key-an*
Cianán *Key-NAWN*
Cianna *Key-ANNA*
Ciar *Kear*
Ciara/keara/kiera/kira *Keyra*
Ciarán *Key-RAWN*
Ciarmhac *KEAR-wac*
Ciarnait *KEAR-nitch*
Cillian *Kill-e-an*
Cillín *Kill -EEN*
Cináed *Kin −AY-ad*
Cinnéide *Kinn-AY-ja*
Cionnaola *Kinn-AY-la*
Clancy *Clan-see*
Clár *Clawr*
Clifden *Cliff-tin*
Clíodhna *CLAY-na*
Clive *Clibe*
Clodagh *CLO-da*
Clothach *CLO-ha*
Clothra *CLO-hra*
Cobhlaith *CO-lee*
Cochrann *CO-hrann*
Cofach *Co-fa*
Coileán *Kill-AWN*
Coilín *Kill-EEN*
Colenso *Co-LEN-so*
Colla *COL-a*
Colm *Colim*
Colmán *Coalman*
Colum *Co-lum*
Columb *Co-lum*
Comhal *Coal*
Conaire *Con-ara*
Conán *Co-NAWN*
Conchobar *CRUH-er*
Conlaodh *Con-LEE*

Conmhac *CON-wac*
Conna *Con-ah*
Connemara *Conn-a-MARA*
Corbally *Corbal-EE*
Corcair *COR-car*
Corcán *Cor-CAWN*
Corcoran *COR-coran*
Corcrán *Cor-CRAWN*
Corentin *COR-entin*
Cormacán *Cor-mac-AWN*
Corrigan *CORIG-an*
Crea *Cray*
Créd *CRAY-ed*
Crinoc *Crin-oc*
Críofán *CREE-FAWN*
Críonán *CREE-NAWN*
Cróchnait *CROKE-nitch*
Croeb *CROW-eb*
Crónán *CROW-NAWN*
Croney *CROW-nee*
Cruinn *Crin*
Cu Chonnacht *Coo Conacht*
Cu Ula *Coo Ala*
Cuán *Coo-AWN*
Cuana *Coo-ANA*
Cúchulainn *COO-chulin*
Cullen *Culin*
Cumhal *COO-wal*
Cumhea *COO-va*
Curragh *Curra*

Dagda *DAG-da*
Dáire *Da-ra*
Daireen *DAR-een*
Dáirine *Dar-EEN-a*
Dáithí *DA-hee*
Dallán *Dal-AWN*
Daman *DA-man*
Damhán *Dav-AWN*
Damhnait *DAV-nitch*

Dana *DA-na*
Danu *DA-noo*
Dara *DA-ra*
Daragh *DA-ra*
Darragh *Dara*
Dary *DA-ree*
Darya *Dar-EE-a*
Davan *DA-van*
Deaglán *JAY-glan*
Deáman *JAH-man*
Dearbháil *DER-vil*
Deargán JAR-gan
Dearlú *JAR-loo*
Decima *De-SEAMA*
Deirdre *DEER-dra*
Delaney *De-LAY-nee*
Delia *DEE-LEE-ah*
Delwen *DEL-wen*
Derbhaíl *Der-vil*
Derryth *Derr-ith*
Dervla *Derv-la*
Dervogilla *Dervo-gila*
Dezi *Dezee*
Dianmitt *JANE-mit*
Diarmaid *DEER-mid*
Docco *DOCK-oh*
Doireann *DER-an*
Dolan *DOUGH-lan*
Donagh *Dona*
Donahue *Dona-who*
Dónal *DOUGH-nal*
Donegal *Dun-ee-gawl*
Donegan *Don-ay-gan*
Donleavy *Dun-LEE-vee*
Donnabhán *Donn-a-VAWN*
Donnagán *Dona-GAWN*
Donnán *Don-AWN*
Donnchadh *Donn-ca*
Donncuan *Don-COON*
Donoghue *Don-AH-who*
Dorian *Doorean*
Dorren *Dorin*
Dowle *Dow-il*
Draigen *Draygin*

Duald *DO-ald*
Dualtach *DOAL-ta*
Duarcan *Dour-can*
Dubh *Doo/Dove*
Dubhán *Doo-AWN/Dove-AWN*
Dubhdara *DOO-dara*
Dubhghall *DOO-gall*
Dubhóg *DOO-vogue*
Dubhthach *DO-ha*
Dufach *Dufa*
Dufferin *Dufferin*
Dugald *DO-gald*
Duibheasa/Duvessa *DOO-vesa*
Duibhleamhna *Div-lowna*
Dúinseach *Doinsha*
Dulane *Dolin*
Dúnlaith *DOON-lee*
Dúnlang *DOON-lang*
Dymphna *Dimph-na*

Eábha *AY-wa*
Eachna *AC-na*
Eachra *AC-ra*
Éachtach *Ac-ta*
Éadaoin *Ay-dean*
Eala *Ala*
Ealga *Alga*
Eamon *Aymon*
Eamonn *Aymon*
Éan *Ian*
Earnán *Ar-NAWN*
Earrach *Ara*
Echlin *Eclin*
Echmhilidh *Ecvilly*
Edern *AY-dern*
Edryd *Edrid*
Eeada *EE-ada*
Egan *Ee-gan*
Eibhear *AYE-vir*
Éibhleann *AYVE-lan*
Eibhlin *EV-lin*
Eilish *Ayelish*
Eilit *EL-itch*
Eiltín *Elt-sheen*

Eilwen *Elwin*
Eily *Ilee*
Eimear *Emer*
Eiméid *EM-edge*
Einín *AY-neen*
Éire *Ayre-a*
Eireamhón *Ara-wone*
Eiros *AIR-os*
Eithne *ETH-na*
Elaina *El-AN-ea*
Eláir *AY-lar*
Elan *AY-lan*
Ellenea *Ellen-EE-a*
Eluned *Elooned*
Emly *Emlee*
Ena *AY-na*
Énán *AY-NAWN*
Enda *EN-da*
Endelient *EN-delient*
Enit *een-it*
Énnae *AY-nay*
Ennis *Enis*
Enog *AY-nog*
Enora *En-AURA*
Enri *EN-ree*
Eny *Any*
Eochaid *O-chid*
Eochaid *O-chee*
Eocho *O-cho*
Eoghan *Owen*
Eoin *Owen*
Eolann *YO-lan*
Epifania *Epee-FANE-ia*
Érne *Airin*
Étaín *AY-TAWN*
Etan *E-tain*
Étaoin *AY-tain*
Eunan *YOU-nan*
Evegren *EVE-gran*
Evena *eh-VEE-nee*
Eveny *ee-veh-nee*

Fachtna *FACT-na*
Faerghus *Fairg-us*
Faife *Fafe*
Faílenn *FEE-len*
Failghe *Fail-ga*

Fainche *Fansha*
Faircheallach *Farcalla*
Faithleann *FIE-lan*
Fallon *Falon*
Fanchea *Fansha*
Faoileann *FWEE-lan*
Faolán *Fay-LAWN*
Farquar *Far-quar*
Farry *FAR-ee*
Feardhach *Fear-ga*
Feardorcha
  Far-DORKA
Feargal *Far-gal*
Fearghal *Far-gal*
Fearghus *Far-gus*
Fedelmid *Fe-DEL-mid*
Feelan *FEE-lan*
Feileacán *Felli-CAWN*
Felim *FAY-lim*
Feothan *Fi-o-han*
Feradach *Ferda*
Féthnat *FAY-nat*
Ffion *Feen*
Fia *Fee-a*
Fiacha *FAY-ca*
Fiachna *FAKE-na*
Fiachra *FAKE-ra*
Fial *Feel*
Fianna *FAY-na*
Fidelma *Fi-DEL-ma*
Filippo *Filipo*
Fimain *Fi-main*
Finbarr *Fin-bar*
Finguine *Fing-wine*
Fínín *Feeneen*
Finin *FIN-in*
Finnabair *Fin-ABAR*
Finnán *Fin-AWN*
Finnbarr *FIN-bar*
Finncháem *Fin-shame*
Finnchnes *Finches*
Finndeach *Finnja*
Finnea *FIN-ay*
Finneacht *Finnacht*
Finnéadan *Finn-AY-dan*
Finnén *Fineen*
Finnguala *Finn-GOO-la*

Finnseach *Finsha*
Fionn *Fin*
Fionnait *Finitch*
Fionnán *Fin-AWN*
Fionntan *Fin-tan*
Fionnúir *Fin-OOR*
Fionnuala *Fin-OO-la*
Fírinne *FEAR-eenya*
Fíthel *Feethel*
Flaherty *FLA-hertee*
Flaithrí *FLY-ree*
Flannait *Flanitch*
Flannán *Flan-AWN*
Flidais *Flidaze*
Fodla *Fola*
Fomhair *For*
Forlaith *Forla*
Fothad *Fohad*
Fráech *Frake*
Fuamnach *FOOM-na*

Gael *Gayle*
Gair *Gar*
Gallagher *Gallaher*
Garbhán *Gar-VAWN*
Gawain *Gawan*
Gealach *Gala*
Gearoíd *Garoyd*
Geiléis *Gaylis*
Geimhreadh *GIV-roo*
Gerwyn *Gerwin*
Gethan *Gehan*
Ginevra *Ginerva*
Giolla *Gila*
Giolla Chriost
  Gila-CREEST
Glaisne *GLASH-na*
Glassán *Glas-AWN*
Glenys *Glenis*
Glorvina *Glor-VEENA*
Glynis *Glinis*
Goilia *GoyLEEa*
Gormlaith *Gormlee*
Gráinne *Grawn-nya*
Grian *Grayan*
Gūaire *Goo-ARA*

Gwynfor *Gwinfour*
Gyleen *GUY-leen*
Gypo *Geepo*

Haco *Haoc*
Haude *Hawid*
Hypathia *High-PAY-theea*
Hywel *Highwel*

Ia *Eea*
Iarom *Earom*
Ibor *Ebor*
Íde *Eeja*
Ifor *Eefor*
Ilaria *Il-AR-ee-a*
Inés *In-ACE*
Inir *In-ir*
Inira *In-ERA*
Inisheer *Inis-ear*
Innis *Inish*
Iodhar *Ear*
Iomhar *Eewar*
Ion *Eon*
Iona *eONA*
Ior *Eeor*
Íosac *Eeosac*
Irial *Ireeal*
Iseult *EE-soolt*
Isibéal *IS-ibel*
Isolde *Eesold*
Isolt *Eesolt*
Ita *Eeta*
Iuchra *Oocra*
Ivan *Ivab*

Jago *Eeago*
Jimeoin *Jim-OWEN*
Jos *Josh*
Juverna *YouVERna*

Kaheena *Ca-HEEN-a*
Kavanagh *Kavna*
Kaylen *KAYlin*
Keir *Care*
Keyne *Kayne*
Killala *Kill-ALA*

Killeigh *Kill-AYE*
Kinsale *Kin-SALE*

Labhaoise *Lou-EE-sha*
Labhraidh *Lowry*
Labhrás *Lowras*
Lachie *Lachee*
Lachtna *Lactna*
Lallóc *La-LOOK*
Lalóg *La-LOOIG*
Laoghaire *Leera*
Laoire *Leera*
Laoise *LEE-sha*
Laoiseach *LEE-sha*
Laragh *Lara*
Lasair *Lasar*
Lasairiona *Lasar-EE-na*
Lasrina *LASreena*
Lassar *Lasare*
Léa *Lee-ah*
Léana *LEE-ana*
Leenane *Lee-NANE*
Lehiff *Lee-HIFF*
Leighlin *LAY-lin*
Lennán *Len-AWN*
Líadaine *Lee-AD-ane*
Líadan *Lee-AD-an*
Líban *LEE-ban*
Líoch *LEE-ach*
Llewellyn *Clewellan*
Loch *Lough*
Lochlainn *Loclan*
Lochlan *Loclan*
Loic *Lick*
Lonergan *Lonergann*
Lonnóg *Lonnogue*
Loughlin *Lochlin*
Lowry *LOW-ree*
Lúcás *LOO-CAWS*
Lucia *LOO-sea-a*
Ludmilla *Lood- ME- la*
Ludovica *Lood-o-VEE-SHA*
Lúgach *LOOG-a*
Lugaid *Louis*
Lugh *Loo*

Lughán *Loo-AWN*
Luíseach *LEE-sha*

MacArdle *Mac AR-dal*
MacBeatha *Mac BA-ha*
MacBirney *Mac BARE-nee*
MacCann *Mac Ann*
MacCarten *Mac AR-tan*
MacCawell *Mac CAW-ell*
MacClosky *Mac CLUSK-ee*
MacClure *Mac LOOR*
MacColum *Mac CO-lim*
MacCoughlin *Mac Cochlin*
MacDarra *Mac Dara*
MacDonagh *Mac Dona*
MacEgan *Mac Eegan*
MacGarry *Mac Gary*
Macha *Maha*
MacKiernan *Mac EARN-an*
MacLoughlin *Mac LOCH-lin*
MacQuade *Mac Wade*
Madeg *MAD-egg*
Madoc *MAD-ock*
Madrun *MAD-roon*
Máen *Main*
Maeve *Maiv*
Magennis *Ma-GIN-is*
Maghera *Mah-ER-a*
Máible *MAY-bla*
Maidie *MAY-dee*
Maik *Mile*
Maille *Mail*
Mailli *Molly*
Mailsi *MAY-lesee*
Mairéad *Maraid*
Máirtin *MART-een*
Majella *Ma-JELLA*
Malachi *Mal-A-key*
Malvina *Mal-VEENA*
Mamie *Mamee*
Manulla *Man-ULLA*

Mánus *MAWN-us*
Manus *Man-us*
Maol Eoin *Mail Owen*
Maol Mhuadh *Mail WOOEY*
Maol Mhuire *Mail Were*
Maolíosa *Mail Eesa*
Maolmhaodhóg *Mail WAYOGUE*
Maolruanal *Mail ROONAL*
Maonach *MAIN-ah*
Marcán *MarCAWN*
Martán *Mar-TAWN*
Maurya *Moura*
Maziere *Ma-ZEER*
Meadhbh *Maev*
Meallán *Mal-AWN*
Medwenna *Mid-WENA*
Mellán *Mel-AWN*
Merewin *Mer-i-win*
Miach *Mia-ac*
Michaeil *MEE-hal*
Midir *Mid-EER*
Milo *MY-low*
Mina *Meena*
Miniver *Mieever*
Moingionn *Mungan*
Molaisse *MO-lass*
Monaghan *MON-a-han*
Monat *Mon-at*
Mondo *Mon-do*
Moninne *Mon-EEN*
Morna *Morn*
Morolt *MORE-olt*
Muadhnait *MOON-itch*
Muchadh *Moocoo*
Mughrón *Mo-RONE*
Muinín *Mwin-EEN*
Muircheartach *Mur-CARTA*
Muireacht *Muract*
Muireann *Mwir-an*
Muirgel *Mwir-gal*
Muírgheal *Mweergal*
Muirgheas *Mwergas*
Muirín *Mwir-EEN*

Muiríos *Mwir-EES*
Muiris *Mwir-ees*
Muirne *Mwirnya*
Murchadh *Murchee*
Murrough *Murah*
Murtagh *Murtah*
Myfanwy *My-FAN-wee*

Naisi *NAY-see*
Naoise *NEE-sha*
Naomh *Neev*
Naomhán *Nee-VAWN*
Nárbhla *NAHR-vla*
Néamh *NEE-ow*
Neamh *Nee-ow*
Neamhain *Nee-OW-an*
Neasa *Nya-SA*
Nechtan *Necktan*
Nehemias *Neh-HE-me-as*
Neilie *Nelly*
Ném *Name*
Nerys *Nerees*
Neve *Neev*
Nevid *NEV-id*
Niall *NIGH-all/ NEE-all*
Niamh *Neev*
Noeleen *NO-leen*
Nona *NO-na*
Nonín *NO-NEEN*
Nuadu *Noo-A-doo*
Nuala *NOO-la*
Nugent *NOO-gent*
Nye *Nie*

O'Beirne *O Bearn*
O'Clery *O CLEAR-ee*
O'Dowd *O Dowid*
O'Herlihy *O HER-li-hee*
O'Lohan *O LOW-han*
O'Loughlin *O LOCH-lan*
O'Molloy *O Mul-oye*
O'Moriarty *O Mor-ee-ARTY*

O'Rourke *O Roarke*
O'Shaughnessy *O SHAWK-ness-ee*
Océane *O-say-an*
Odhrán *Or-an*
Óengus *Aing-gus*
Ogilvy *O-gil-vee*
Oisín *O-sheen*
Oistin *Aus-tin*
Olwen *Ol-wen*
Omagh *O-ma*
Ónait *O-nitch*
Onilwyn *O-nil-win*
Oola *OO-la*
Oona *OO-na*
Órán *O-RAWN*
Oran *O-ran*
Orinthia *O-RIN-thee-a*
Órla *OR-la*
Órlaith *OR-lee*
Osnait *Os-nitch*
Owny *O-wen-ee*

Pádraic *PAW-ric*
Pádraig *PAW-drig*
Pádraigín *PAW-drig-EEN*
Paili *Palee*
Pallas *Palas*
Patsy *PAT-see*
Paudeen *PAW-deen*
Peadar *Pah-der*
Pegeen *Pegeen*
Peig *Peg*
Penwyn *PEN-win*
Petroc *Pet-rock*
Phelan *FAY-lan*
Phelim *FAY-lim*
Philomena *Filomeena*
Philpog *FILP-ogue*
Piala *PEE-A-la*
Pilib *Pilib*
Póilín *PO-leen*

Rahan *RA-han*
Ráichéal *RAYTCH-el*
Raina *RAIN-a*

Ramoan *RAH-moan*
Ranalt *RAN-alt*
Réalta *Rayalta*
Realtán *Rail-TAWN*
Réamonn *RAY-mon*
Reardan *RAYAR-dan*
Rhain *Rain*
Rhedyn *RAY-deen*
Rhian *Reean*
Rhianwen *Ree-AN-when*
Rhonwen *Ron-when*
Rhydach *Rie-dack*
Rhydwyn *Rie-dwin*
Rían *Reean*
Rina *Reena*
Riona *Ree-o-na*
Ríonach *Reena*
Riordan *REAR-dan*
Roche *Rotche*
Rodán *ROE-DAWN*
Roden *ROE-den*
Rohan *ROE-han*
Rois *Royce*
Róisín *RO-sheen*
Romy *ROME-ee*
Rónait *ROAN-itch*
Rónal *ROAN-al*
Ronan *ROAN-an*
Roone *Roon*
Rós *ROE-ish*
Rozenn *ROZ-en*
Rúadhán *ROO-AWN*
Ruaidhri *Ruir-EE*
Rumann *RUM-an*
Rumo *ROOM-o*
Rumon *ROO--mon*

Sadb/Sadbh *Saiv/Sive*
Saibreas *SEV-ris*
Samhaoir *SA-weir*
Samhradh *SOW-roo*
Saoirse *SAYOR-sha*
Sárait *Saw-ritch*
Sawyer *SAW-yer*
Scannlán *Scann-lan*
Scathach *Sca-ha*

Scáthach *Sca-ha*
Sciath *Skayah*
Scota *Scot-ah*
Scoth *Scoh*
Séadach *SHAY-da*
Seafra *SHAF-ra*
Seagrun *SHAY-groon*
Seanán *SHAN-AWN*
Seanchen *SHAN-cen*
Séarlait *SHAR-lit*
Séimi *SHAY-me*
Seirian *Sher-ian*
Senan *Sen-ann*
Seodra *Show-dra*
Sererena *Sir-er-EENA*
Sergius *Ser-GEE-us*
Seumas *Shaymus*
Seva *SAY-va*
Shamus *SHAY-mus*
Shanahan *SHAN-ah-han*
Shasta *SHAS-ta*
Shaun *Shone*
Shauna *SHONE-a*
Shay *Shay*
Shea *Shay*
Sheridan *SHARE-id-an*
Shiby *Shibee*
Sholeh *SHOW-lay*
Sian *SEE-an*
Sibéal *Sib-ale*
Síle *SHEE-la*
Sillán *Sill-AWN*
Sinead *SHIN-aid*
Siobhan *SHIV-aun*
Síocháin *SHE-CAWN*
Síoda *She-ADA*
Siollán *Shil-AWN*
Siomha *She-wa*
Sitric *Sit-rick*
Siún *Shoe-an*
Sive *SIGH-ve*
Skia *Ski-a*

Sláine *SLAYN-a*
Sligo *SLY-go*
Solam *SO-lam*
Sorcha *SOR-ca*
Sorley *SOR-lee*
Spéir *Spare*
Standish *STAN-dish*
Stébhín *STAY-veen*
Stiofán *Sti-FAWN*
Strachan *SRACK-an*
Suanach *SOON-a*
Suibne *Siv-ne*
Suir *Soor*
Sulian *Soolian*

Tailbreamh *Tile-brew*
Taillte *Tall-cha*
Taliesin *Tall-is-in*
Tallis *Tal-is*
Tancredi *Tank-RAY-dee*
Tangi *Tang-ee*
Tanguy *Tan-guy*
Tárlach *TAAR-la*
Teagan *Tay-gan*
Teague *Taid*
Teámhair *TAY-war*
Tegwen *Teg-wen*
Teigue *Taig*
Teimhnín *Tev-NEEN*
Temair *TAY-mar*
Tempo *Tem-po*
Thadóir *Thadore*
Thalia *Thal-EE-a*
Tiaquin *Te-a-quin*
Tiarnach *Cheerna*
Tiarnán *Cheer-NAWN*
Tibbot *Tib-ot*
Tibor *TEE-bor*
Tiernan *CHEER-nan*
Tierney *CHEER-nee*
Tirian *CHEER-ee-an*
Toimilin *Tom-il-in*
Tomaltach *Tom-AL-ta*

Tomás *To-MASS*
Torin *Tor-in*
Tralee *Tra-LEE*
Tremaine *TRAY-main*
Tremayne *TRAY-main*
Trevelyan *Trev-el-ian*
Triona *Treena*
Tuathal *TOO-hal*
Tuathla *TOO-hla*
Tuilelath *Tilla-la*
Tynan *TIE-nan*
Tyrella *TIE-rella*
Tyrrell *TIE-rel*

Uainionn *Ooanin*
Uaithne *Oo-ITHNE*
Uallach *Oo-LAH*
Ualtar *Oo-al-tar*
Ughaire *Oo-JARA*
Uilleag *Ill-yig*
Uilliam *Ill-iam*
Uinseann *Inshin*
Una *Oo-na*
Úna *OO-na*
Urien *YOUR-ian*
Urquhart *Ur-quart*

Vartry *Vart-tree*
Vaughan *Vawn*
Vevina *Vev-EENA*
Visant *Vighsant*

Wenn *When*

Xenia *Zeenia*

Yestin *YEST-in*
Ynyr *EEN-er*

Zaira *Sa-REE-a*
Zarah *Zara*
Zinna *ZEE-na*
Zozim *SOS-eem*

Index

Faílenn 77, 94, 105
Failghe 122, 123
Fainche 77, 105, 112
Faircheallach 108
Faithleann 108
Fallon 17, 108
family names
    115–26
famous names 31–65
Fanchea 105
Fann 77
Faoileann 105
Faolán 100, 108, 110
Farquar 24
Farrell 17, 120, 121,
    122
Farrell, Colin 34
Farrelly 108
Farry 13
Fay 152
Faye 7
Feardhach 119
Feardorcha 13
Feargal 35
Fearghal 126
Fearghus 108
Fedelmid 87
Federica 27
Feelan 105
Feileacán 146
Felim 100
Felix 28
Feothan 146
Feradach 124
Fergal 150
Fergus 23, 55, 87,
    100, 108
Ferguson 24
Féthnat 77
Ffion 20
Fia 146
Fiacha 117, 122, 125
Fiachna 87
Fiachra 153
Fial 77
Fianna 47
Fidelma 77, 105
Fife 24
Filippo 28
Fimain 148
Finbar 59
Finbarr 108
Finch 55
Finguine 101, 124
Finin 119, 125, 126

Finlay 10, 153
Finley 10, 39
Finn xi, 14, 39–40,
    51, 59, 69, 70, 87,
    122, 123, 130, 153
Finnabair 78
Finnán 108
Finnbarr 14, 58
Finncháem 78
Finnchnes 78
Finndeach 14
Finnea 130
Finneacht 14, 94
Finnéadan 14
Finnegan 14, 136
Finnén 108
Finnguala 78
Finnian 14
Finnigan 40
Finnoola 54
Finnseach 14
Finola 14, 116, 117
Fintan 14, 35, 108,
    110
Fiona 14, 35, 40, 59,
    105, 148, 152
Fionn xi, 4, 8, 87,
    153
Fionnait 105
Fionnán 108
Fionntan 108, 110
Fionnuala 14, 64, 78
    116, 148
Fionnúir 14
Fionnula 35
Fírinne 146, 148
Fíthel 87
Fitzgerald 118
Fitzgerald, Orla 35
Flaherty 136
Flaithrí 101
Flanagan 15, 17, 136
Flanagan, Fionnula
    35
Flann 15, 17, 94,
    101, 108
Flannait 15
Flannán 15, 108
Flannery 15
Flavie 27
Flidais 78
Flockhart, Calista 41
Flora 27, 105
Florence 119
Florrie 143

Flurry 144
Flynn 15, 17, 40, 59,
    136, 153
Fodla 78
Foley 118
Fomhair 146
Forbes 24
Forlaith 94
Fothad 123
Fráech 88
Francesca 27
Fraser 24
Freddy 144, 153
Frederick 119
Frost, Sadie 42
Fuamnach 78
Fyfe 24

Gabriel 51
Gael 88
Gaia 27
Gair 24
Gallagher 136
Gallagher, Cathal 34
Gallagher, Liam 41,
    44
Gallagher, Noel 39,
    44
Gallagher, Rory 36
Galway 130
Garbhán 108
Gareth (female) 59
Gareth 24, 153
Garrett 51
Garrett-Michael 122
Garth, Jenny 40
Garvin 108
Gawain 24
Gay 35
Gaynor 20
Gealach 146
Gearoíd 113, 118
Geiléis 148
Geimhreadh 146
Gemma 59
Gene 44
George 65
Georgie 144
Gerry 64
Gerwyn 24
Gethan 20
Gianna 27
Gilkevin 126
Gill 118
Gilligan 136

Ginevra 27
Giolla 112
Giolla Chriost 119
girls' names 5, 6, 7, 9,
    10, 13, 14, 15,
    16–17, 18–21,
    27–8, 34–6, 50–1,
    53–4, 64, 71–82,
    91–6, 105–6,
    111–12, 116–17,
    142–3, 147–9,
    151–2
Glaisne 120, 121,
    126
Glas 88
Glassán 101
Glenny 118
Glenys 20
Glin 130
Gloria 54, 62
Glorvina 54, 62
Glyn 24
Glynis 20
Goilia 119
Gorman 14, 17, 101,
    124
Gormlaith 94
Grace 5, 7, 44, 152
Gracie 143
Graham 24
Gráinne x, 70, 78,
    94–5, 112, 115,
    116, 117, 152
Grania 116, 117
Gregor 24
Grian 79, 148
Griffin 107, 118
Griffith 24
Guaire 101
Guggi 44
Gulliver 40
Gus 144
Guthrie 24
Gwanwen 20
Gwen 20
Gwyneth 20
Gwynfor 24
Gyleen 130
Gypo 48

Haco 24
Hamilton, Scott 37
Hamish 24
Hannah 5
Harriet 152

About the Authors

PAMELA REDMOND SATRAN is a contributing editor for *Parenting* magazine and a columnist for *Glamour*. She is the author of five novels, including *The Man I Should Have Married,* and writes frequently for publications including *The New York Times* and *The Huffington Post*. She lives outside New York City with her husband and three children.

LINDA ROSENKRANTZ is the author of seven other books in addition to the baby-naming series, ranging from *Gone Hollywood,* a social history of the film colony; to a childhood memoir, *My Life as a List: 207 Things About My (Bronx) Childhood;* to a history and anthology of telegrams. A resident of Los Angeles, she also writes a syndicated weekly column on collectibles.

As authorities on baby names, they have been quoted in *People,* the *Wall Street Journal,* and the *New York Times Magazine*. They have also made appearances on nationally syndicated shows such as *Oprah* and the CNN Morning News. Their baby-name books have sold more than one million copies. Find them on the web at www.nameberry.co.uk.